Mortality statistics

perinatal and infant: social and biological factors

Review of the Registrar General
on deaths in England and Wales,
1986

Series DH3 no. 20

London: Her Majesty's Stationery Office

ISBN 0 11 691245 6

Contents

Cause of death   England and Wales

Numbers of previous stillbirths (legitimate only)   England and Wales

Duration of pregnancy   England and Wales

Birthweight   England and Wales
Numbers and rates per 1,000 total/live births

Place of confinement, age of mother and legitimacy   England and Wales

Month of birth   England and Wales

Multiple births   England and Wales

Introduction

Mortality statistics: perinatal and infant (social and biological factors) 1986 deals with statistics produced from stillbirth records and from the linkage of infant death records to their corresponding birth records. Comparable statistics for 1975 to 1985 have been published elsewhere.[1-8]

Since 1975 infant death records have been linked to their corresponding birth records in order to obtain information on the social and biological factors of the baby's family. Only a limited amount of information (some of which is confidential) relating to the parents of the deceased infant is obtainable from death registration but a considerable amount of information (including confidential particulars) is given at birth registration, including age of parents, number of previous legitimate children (parity), occupation of parent (usually father), country of birth of parents, institution of birth and whether the baby was a singleton or not. This report presents data on all these factors and also includes information on cause of death, region of residence, and birthweight.

Deaths of infants have been separated into five groups which are not mutually exclusive: stillbirths, perinatal deaths (stillbirths and deaths occurring in the first week of life), neonatal deaths (occurring in the first four weeks of life), postneonatal deaths (occurring from the fifth week of life up to one year of age) and infant deaths (occurring in the first year of life).

In the majority of the analyses illegitimate births have been treated separately. One reason for this is that the mother's parity is not included in the information given at the registration of an illegitimate birth. In addition, the occupation data available for illegitimate births are based on the mother's occupation unless the birth was registered jointly by the father and the mother. (In 1986, 66 per cent of illegitimate births were registered jointly.) Thus for illegitimate children registered by the mother alone, only the social class of the mother is available. This information is not comparable with that obtained for legitimate births.

Stillbirths and neonatal deaths - changes to cause of death coding in 1986

On 1 January 1986 new stillbirth and neonatal death certificates were introduced in England and Wales. These certificates follow the recommendations of the World Health Organisation made in the 9th Revision of the *International Classification of Diseases* whereby the causes of death are given separately in the following categories:

a) Main diseases or conditions in fetus or infant
b) Other diseases or conditions in fetus or infant
c) Main maternal diseases or conditions affecting fetus or infant
d) Other maternal diseases or conditions affecting fetus or infant
e) Other relevant causes.

Whilst conditions arising in the mother which affected the fetus or infant could be mentioned on the old certificates, no provision was made for those cases in which the doctor thought that both maternal and fetal conditions contributed equally to the death. The new certificates overcome this problem. However, since equal weighting is given to main conditions in the fetus and in the mother, it is no longer possible to identify a single underlying cause of death for stillbirths and neonatal deaths. Therefore all tabulations which include cause have had to be re-designed and now include the total number of mentioned conditions. It should be noted that a baby can have more than one main fetal condition and more than one main maternal condition.

Further work is being undertaken to evaluate the best means of presenting the data.

Methods of study

A computer aided system enables annual production of linked data. Linking is achieved by using the National Health Service (NHS) number of the dead child to identify the birth registration. Briefly, the system is as follows: draft entries of deaths (which are forms completed by the local registrar from information supplied during the interview with the informant) are sent to the NHS Central Register so that the Register can be updated. Drafts relating to children under one year of age are separated and the NHS number is entered (if not already present).

Drafts relating to children born abroad, dead foundlings, or adopted children are removed (for a child born abroad or a dead foundling there is no birth registration available and linkage is not permissible in the case of an adopted child). These drafts along with any others that failed to be linked have been analysed separately (see next section).

Identification information from the death drafts is then entered on a magnetic tape record and matched by computer to a file of all infant deaths, previously extracted from the annual file of records of all deaths in England and Wales, enabling the enhancement of these records with the

NHS number. The automated system checks that all drafts relating to deaths of infants under one year of age have been extracted; any records on the computer file or among the set of drafts which are not matched with another record are listed for clerical scrutiny. The death record enhanced with the NHS number is then linked to the birth record. The NHS number is derived from birth registration information and is therefore available on the birth record. The criteria used to decide that a correct link has occurred are the NHS number, date of birth and sex of the child. Queries are resolved clerically. The final stage is the merging of linked records with stillbirth records (which are complete in themselves) to produce a computer file for tabulations.

Linkage of infant death records to their corresponding birth records enables production of two types of data file, one being the traditional type of infant mortality data (deaths registered in a calendar year), and the other a birth cohort with the data relating to deaths among children born in a calendar year. Most of the tabulations are of the traditional type and present statistics for deaths registered in 1986; the only exceptions are the one by month of birth and those for multiple births. These latter tabulations present statistics for deaths occurring to babies born in 1985 because the birth cohort data for a given year do not become available until a year after the traditional type of data.

For infant mortality, the two types of data files differ very little, as over half of the infant deaths occur in the first week of life and two thirds occur in the first month, with the result that almost all the deaths occur in the same year as the birth. The difference will be greater for postneonatal mortality where more children may die in the calendar year following their birth. There will, however, only be a difference in the mortality rates obtained from the two types of data if there is a large fluctuation in the number of births or a rapid change in the underlying mortality rates.

Analysis of unlinked cases

Table A shows the linkage rate for infant deaths for each of the four years 1983 to 1986, and the reasons why the records failed to link. The linkage rate, which remained at 98.5 per cent in 1983 and 1984, then fell to 98.1 per cent in 1985, then rose again in 1986 to 98.4 per cent.

The unlinked cases can be split into two groups; those which cannot be linked (such as those born outside England and Wales, dead foundlings and adopted children) and others which theoretically should have been linked. The percentage of deaths in this second category fell steadily from 1975 when linkage began (when they formed 0.9 per cent of all deaths) to a low of 0.2 per cent in 1980. This proportion has remained at 0.2 or 0.3 since then.

General Notes

Social class

In this volume, only deaths of legitimate infants have been analysed by social class, due to differences in the recording of occupational data for parents of infants born illegitimate described previously. The social class of a child born legitimate is taken as the social class of the child's father: this has been derived from the father's occupation and status (for example, whether or not he is a foreman) as recorded at birth registration.

For 1986 data, the *1980 Classification of Occupations*[9] has been used. The social class categories used are:

Social Class I Professional occupations (for example doctors and lawyers)
Social Class II Intermediate occupations (for example teachers and managers)

Table A Linkage rate 1983 to 1986

	1983		1984		1985		1986	
	Number	Per cent	Number	Per cent	Number	Per cent	Number	Per cent
All infant deaths	**6,381**	**100.0**	**6,037**	**100.0**	**6,141**	**100.0**	**6,313**	**100.0**
Linked infant deaths	6,284	98.5	5,945	98.5	6,027	98.1	6,209	98.4
Unlinked infant deaths								
Cannot be linked	78	1.2	77	1.3	95	1.5	86	1.4
Should have been linked	19	0.3	15	0.2	19	0.3	18	0.3
All unlinked cases	**97**	**100.0**	**92**	**100.0**	**114**	**100.0**	**104**	**100.0**
Born outside England and Wales	72	74.2	61	66.3	71	62.3	54	51.9
Adopted child	1	1.0	-	-	-	-	-	-
Foundling	5	5.2	16	17.4	18	15.8	9	8.7
No trace of birth record	17	17.5	10	10.9	15	13.2	18	17.3
Miscellaneous	2	2.1	5	5.4	10	8.8	23	22.1

Social Class IIIN Non-manual skilled occupations (for example clerks and shop assistants)
Social Class IIIM Manual skilled occupations (for example bricklayers and underground coalminers)
Social Class IV Partly skilled occupations (for example bus conductors and postmen)
Social Class V Unskilled occupations (for example porters and labourers)
Other This includes residual groups, such as armed forces, persons with inadequately described occupations, persons who were unoccupied and persons with no stated occupation, who are not assigned to Social Classes I to V.

Legitimacy

Since some infants are legitimated between birth and death, the 'true' illegitimate infant mortality rate, which relates those infants dying in the first year of life who were born illegitimate with the number of illegitimate live births, can only be produced when the infant death record has been linked to the corresponding birth record. In this volume all tabulations of legitimacy relate to legitimacy at birth.

Parity

Information on previous children is only available for women having a legitimate birth. In this volume, parity is defined as the number of previous live or still born children by the present or any former husband, as stated at birth registration.

Area of residence

Table 7 shows data by regional health authority of residence of mother at the time of the child's death. These data relate to the RHAs as they have existed since the re-organisation of the health service which was implemented in April 1982. Infant deaths where the area of usual residence of the mother was outside England and Wales are included in the total figures for England and Wales but excluded from any sub-division of England and Wales.

Information about the place of birth of the parents of children born in England and Wales has been recorded at birth registration since 1969, but data relating to the birthplace of parents have only been available for an infant mortality study of social factors since 1975 when routine linkage was started. It is important to remember, when interpreting these data, that birthplace does not necessarily indicate ethnic origin or race. For example, there are women born in India, whose fathers were there in the civil service, in the armed forces or in business and who later returned to Britain, and these women are now in the childbearing age-groups. Their children will be included in the groups shown as 'mother born in New Commonwealth or Pakistan' although they are not of Indian or Pakistani ethnic origin. Also there is an increasing number of young mothers who were born in Britain but whose parents are of New Commonwealth or Pakistani ethnic origin. In this

volume these mothers are not identifiable among the groups of UK-born residents. For a discussion of this problem see 'New Commonwealth and Pakistani population estimates' in *Population Trends 9*[10] and 'Estimating the size of the ethnic minority populations in the 1980s' in *Population Trends 44*[11].

Birthweight

Information on birthweight for live births has been made available to the Office of Population Censuses and Surveys (OPCS) since 1975 by the co-operation of district medical officers who have been transferring the birthweight, obtained via the birth notification system, to local registrars who copy it on to the birth draft entry forms. These are then forwarded to OPCS for statistical processing. A similar system operates for stillbirths although the initial souce of the information is the medical certificate which is prepared by the certifying doctor and is passed, usually by the parent, to the registrar. This system has been showing consistent improvement in the levels of birthweight recording; in 1977 under 60 per cent of live birth draft entry forms had a recorded birthweight, by 1980 just under 90 per cent had a recorded birthweight, and in 1986 birthweight recording levels were 99.9 per cent for livebirths and 99.2 per cent for stillbirths.

Causes of death

The data have been classified according to the *International Classification of Diseases, Injuries and Causes of Death, 1975* Ninth Revision (ICD)[12] which came into operation at the beginning of 1979.

OPCS has assigned both ICD Eighth Revision and ICD Ninth Revision codes to 25 per cent of all deaths in 1978 as a bridge-coding exercise, the results of which give a guide to the effect of the new classification on specific categories[13,14].

The causes shown in tables of postneonatal deaths are selected causes and therefore the individual categories may not add to the total, while those shown in tables of stillbirths and neonatal deaths are grouped categories which include all ICD codes mentioned on the certificate. **Appendix A** shows N-list numbers with associated descriptions and ICD codes.

Place of confinement

Five categories are used in the tabulation of place of confinement:

NHS hospital A - hospitals and homes under the National Health Service (except psychiatric hospitals) with beds allocated to GP maternity but without a consultant obstetric unit.
NHS hospital B - hospitals and homes under the National Health Service (except psychiatric hospitals) with a consultant obstetric unit. Some hospitals in this category also have GP maternity beds.

Other hospitals - mainly maternity homes not under the National Health Service.

At home - at the usual place of residence of the mother.

Elsewhere - includes all psychiatric institutions, homes for unmarried mothers, remand homes, reception centres, private houses (other than mother's usual residence).

Multiple Births

Information relating to maternities resulting in multiple deliveries is given in **Tables 31** and **32**. It should be noted that these data may represent an underenumeration of the numbers of multiple pregnancies. If a multiple delivery occurs before 28 weeks of gestation and includes both live and dead fetuses, only the live births can be registered under current registration practice.

Definitions

Stillbirths	late fetal deaths: after 28 weeks of gestation	rates per thousand live and still births
Perinatal deaths	stillbirths, and deaths in the first week of life	

Early neonatal deaths	deaths in the first 6 days of life	
Late neonatal deaths	deaths at ages 7-27 completed days of life	rates per thousand live births
Postneonatal deaths	deaths at ages 28 days and over but under one year	
Infant deaths	deaths at ages under one year	

Tabulation and analyses

The tabulations are in five main and several small sections, each presenting data on a particular characteristic of the child's birth or death, or of its parents. The five main sections are: social class, region of residence, country of birth of parents, cause of death and birthweight. Information on social class is also contained in the region of residence, cause of death and birthweight sections. All the main sections contain a breakdown by age at death and by mother's age and by parity and/or legitimacy. Detailed analysis by mother's age and parity is contained in the first section on social class. The other sections present data on number of previous stillbirths, duration of pregnancy, place of confinement, month of birth and multiple births.

The detailed tabulations enable users to produce grouped categories of data, relating to both numbers and rates.

Symbols and conventions used

0.0, 0.00   less than 0.05, 0.005 respectively

-          nil

..   not available or not appropriate

Rates calculated from less than 20 deaths or stillbirths are printed in italics as a warning to the user that their reliability as a measure may be affected by the small number of events.

Changes in 1978

On 1 January 1978 certain provisions of the Criminal Law Act 1977, the Coroners (Amendment) Rules 1977 and the Registration of Births, Deaths and Marriages (Amendment) Regulations 1977 came into force. The two principal changes arising out of the legislation are (a) the abolition of the duty of a coroner's jury to name a person it finds guilty of causing a death and of a coroner to commit that person for trial and (b) in the case where an inquest is adjourned because a person has been charged with an offence in connection with the death, the introduction of provision for the death to be registered at the time of adjournment instead of, as previously, having to await the outcome of the criminal proceedings. The result of such proceedings is notified by the coroner at a later date.

This legislation has a small but significant effect in the compilation of mortality statistics from accidental or violent causes. As recommended in the ICD[12], all deaths assigned to these causes are coded in two ways, to nature of injury codes and to external cause of injury (E) codes. It is not possible to assign the correct E code to some of these accelerated registration cases until results of proceedings are known.

Accordingly, the following procedures have been adopted. The E categories which are most affected by the legislation are those relating to motor vehicle incidents, homocides and open verdicts. From January 1978 all accelerated registrations relating to traffic incidents are coded to the appropriate traffic accident, as sufficient data are available on the coroner's certificate of adjournment. All other accelerated registrations are assigned to E988 (injury by other and unspecified means, undetermined whether accidentally or purposely inflicted) until results of proceedings are known and the death can be reassigned to the correct E code.

When statistics were compiled for 1986 there were 297 deaths assigned to E988 still awaiting results of proceedings.

References

1. Adelstein A M, Macdonald Davies I M, Weatherall J A C. Perinatal and infant mortality: social and bio logical factors 1975-77. *Studies on Medical and Population Subjects* No.41. HMSO (1980).

2. *Mortality statistics: perinatal and infant (social and biological factors) 1978, 1979.* Series DH3 no.7. HMSO (1982).

3. *Mortality statistics: perinatal and infant (social and biological factors) 1980* Series DH3 no.9. HMSO (1983).

4. *Mortality statistics: perinatal and infant (social and biological factors) 1981* Series DH3 no.13. HMSO (1985).

5. *Mortality statistics: perinatal and infant (social and biological factors) 1982* Series DH3 no.14. HMSO (1985).

6. *Mortality statistics: perinatal and infant (social and biological factors) 1983* Series DH3 no.15. HMSO (1986).

7. *Mortality statistics: perinatal and infant (social and biological factors) 1984* Series DH3 no.17. HMSO (1986).

8. *Mortality statistics: perinatal and infant (social and biological factors) 1985* Series DH3 no.18. HMSO (1987).

9. *Classification of Occupations, 1980.* HMSO (1980).

10. OPCS Immigrant Statistics Unit. New Common wealth and Pakistani population estimates. *Population Trends 9.* HMSO (1977).

11. OPCS Population Statistics Division. Estimating the size of the ethnic minority populations in the 1980s. *Population Trends 44.* HMSO (1986).

12. *International Classification of Diseases, Injuries and Causes of Death, 1975* - Ninth Revision. WHO (1977).

13. *OPCS Monitor* DH1 81/82. Bridge-coding 1978: 8th/9th Revision ICD. OPCS (1981).

14. *Mortality statistics: comparison of 8th and 9th Revisions of the International Classification of Diseases, 1978 (sample).* Series DH1 no.10. HMSO (1983).

Table 1 Stillbirths - numbers and rates per 1,000 total births: age of mother x parity, social class (legitimate only); 1986   **England and Wales**

Parity	Social class	Age of mother											
		All ages		Under 20		20 - 24		25 - 29		30 - 34		35 and over	
		Number	Rate	Number	Rate	Number	Rate	Number	Rate	Number	Rate	Number	Rate
All		3,549	5.3	367	6.4	1,017	5.3	1,098	4.8	680	5.2	387	7.2
All legitimate	All	2,600	5.0	107	6.0	668	4.8	907	4.5	581	5.0	337	7.2
	I-V	2,439	4.9	97	5.9	611	4.7	843	4.4	561	4.9	327	7.2
	I	150	3.7	-	-	15	3.8	56	3.5	48	3.3	31	5.1
	II	478	4.0	5	4.2	66	3.6	178	3.8	146	3.9	83	5.2
	IIIN	267	4.8	10	8.6	63	5.0	102	4.2	67	5.1	25	5.3
	IIIM	939	5.2	37	5.3	263	4.7	339	4.7	183	5.3	117	9.5
	IV	419	5.7	23	5.3	135	4.9	125	4.8	86	7.7	50	10.9
	V	186	6.6	22	8.6	69	5.8	43	4.8	31	9.7	21	12.0
	Others	161	6.7	10	6.9	57	6.2	64	7.4	20	5.7	10	8.1
0	All	1,141	5.5	88	6.3	411	5.5	411	5.2	155	5.1	76	9.1
	I-V	1,057	5.4	79	6.2	372	5.3	386	5.1	148	5.0	72	8.9
	I	75	4.4	-	-	12	4.6	37	4.3	17	3.8	9	7.3
	II	208	4.2	5	4.8	47	4.0	82	3.7	51	4.6	23	7.3
	IIIN	135	5.6	9	9.8	38	4.9	64	6.0	18	4.8	6	5.3
	IIIM	396	5.8	32	5.9	160	5.5	142	5.7	36	4.8	26	13.6
	IV	168	6.1	19	5.9	74	5.5	47	5.8	22	9.5	6	11.1
	V	75	8.1	14	7.4	41	8.5	14	7.1	4	8.1	2	13.5
	Others	84	7.9	9	7.3	39	7.7	25	8.1	7	7.2	4	15.5
1	All	731	3.9	16	4.3	177	3.7	281	3.6	183	4.0	74	5.5
	I-V	690	3.8	15	4.3	163	3.7	262	3.5	178	4.0	72	5.5
	I	48	3.1	-	-	3	2.3	16	2.7	19	3.0	10	4.7
	II	151	3.4	-	-	13	2.5	59	3.2	52	3.3	27	5.2
	IIIN	73	3.5	1	4.2	20	5.1	24	2.5	23	4.3	5	3.2
	IIIM	266	4.0	4	2.9	70	3.5	115	4.0	59	4.8	18	5.8
	IV	110	4.5	3	2.9	40	4.2	38	4.0	18	5.2	11	11.1
	V	42	4.5	7	11.7	17	3.6	10	3.4	7	9.5	1	4.8
	Others	41	4.8	1	4.9	14	4.4	19	5.6	5	3.7	2	5.6
2	All	403	4.9	3	9.8	54	4.2	133	4.3	135	5.2	78	6.5
	I-V	378	4.8	3	10.4	51	4.2	119	4.1	130	5.2	75	6.3
	I	18	3.1	-	..	-	-	3	2.2	9	3.3	6	3.7
	II	82	4.4	-	-	4	3.5	26	4.7	32	4.3	20	4.4
	IIIN	40	5.3	-	-	5	6.5	9	3.1	17	6.0	9	8.5
	IIIM	150	5.2	1	8.4	22	4.4	50	4.1	49	5.7	28	8.7
	IV	58	4.7	1	16.7	13	3.9	20	3.9	16	5.6	8	7.9
	V	30	5.6	1	12.6	7	3.7	11	4.9	7	9.0	4	10.1
	Others	25	7.9	-	-	3	4.0	14	8.9	5	8.6	3	11.7
3 and over	All	325	7.3	-	-	26	8.0	82	6.1	108	7.2	109	8.7
	I-V	314	7.3	-	-	25	8.0	76	5.9	105	7.3	108	8.9
	I	9	3.7	-	..	-	-	-	-	3	3.0	6	5.5
	II	37	5.0	-	..	2	8.4	11	7.8	11	4.0	13	4.3
	IIIN	19	6.6	-	..	-	-	5	6.6	9	8.1	5	5.4
	IIIM	127	7.5	-	-	11	7.9	32	5.7	39	6.7	45	11.1
	IV	83	9.6	-	-	8	8.8	20	6.5	30	11.5	25	12.2
	V	39	8.9	-	-	4	8.2	8	4.7	13	10.8	14	14.0
	Others	11	6.6	-	..	1	8.4	6	10.4	3	4.8	1	2.8
Illegitimate		949	6.7	260	6.5	349	6.4	191	6.8	99	7.5	50	7.3

Table 2 Perinatal deaths - numbers and rates per 1,000 total births: age of mother x parity, social class (legitimate only); 1986 — **England and Wales**

Parity	Social class	Age of mother All ages		Under 20		20 - 24		25 - 29		30 - 34		35 and over	
		Number	Rate	Number	Rate	Number	Rate	Number	Rate	Number	Rate	Number	Rate
All		**6,338**	**9.5**	**728**	**12.6**	**1,823**	**9.4**	**1,948**	**8.5**	**1,172**	**9.0**	**667**	**12.5**
All legitimate	All	**4,591**	**8.8**	190	10.6	1,188	8.6	1,630	8.1	1,012	8.7	571	12.3
	I-V	**4,286**	**8.6**	167	10.2	1,087	8.4	1,512	7.8	976	8.6	544	12.0
	I	**293**	**7.2**	1	4.3	25	6.3	113	7.0	94	6.5	60	9.9
	II	**865**	**7.2**	9	7.5	123	6.7	345	7.3	249	6.7	139	8.7
	IIIN	**465**	**8.4**	15	12.9	104	8.3	174	7.2	129	9.9	43	9.2
	IIIM	**1,611**	**8.9**	71	10.2	468	8.4	574	8.0	311	9.1	187	15.2
	IV	**729**	**9.9**	40	9.3	246	9.0	220	8.5	143	12.7	80	17.5
	V	**323**	**11.4**	31	12.1	121	10.1	86	9.7	50	15.6	35	20.0
	Others	**305**	**12.7**	23	15.8	101	11.1	118	13.7	36	10.2	27	22.0
0	All	**1,971**	**9.5**	151	10.9	690	9.2	712	9.0	295	9.6	123	14.7
	I-V	**1,825**	**9.3**	131	10.4	625	9.0	671	8.8	283	9.5	115	14.2
	I	**128**	**7.5**	-	-	19	7.3	61	7.1	34	7.5	14	11.3
	II	**373**	**7.6**	9	8.7	77	6.6	168	7.6	83	7.4	36	11.4
	IIIN	**217**	**9.0**	14	15.3	59	7.6	91	8.5	42	11.2	11	9.8
	IIIM	**693**	**10.1**	56	10.3	278	9.5	242	9.8	80	10.8	37	19.4
	IV	**300**	**10.9**	33	10.3	134	10.0	83	10.2	37	15.9	13	24.0
	V	**114**	**12.3**	19	10.1	58	12.1	26	13.2	7	14.2	4	27.0
	Others	**146**	**13.8**	20	16.2	65	12.9	41	13.2	12	12.3	8	31.1
1	All	**1,379**	**7.3**	33	9.0	340	7.1	548	6.9	319	7.0	139	10.3
	I-V	**1,293**	**7.2**	30	8.6	315	7.1	505	6.7	310	7.0	133	10.1
	I	**98**	**6.3**	1	-14.0	6	4.6	40	6.9	33	5.2	18	8.5
	II	**289**	**6.5**	-	-	32	6.2	120	6.6	89	5.6	48	9.3
	IIIN	**157**	**7.5**	1	4.2	39	9.9	58	5.9	46	8.6	13	8.3
	IIIM	**472**	**7.2**	13	9.4	129	6.5	193	6.6	99	8.1	38	12.1
	IV	**203**	**8.2**	6	5.7	74	7.7	77	8.0	32	9.3	14	14.2
	V	**74**	**8.0**	9	15.0	35	7.4	17	5.7	11	15.0	2	9.6
	Others	**86**	**10.1**	3	14.6	25	7.8	43	12.7	9	6.7	6	16.8
2	All	**697**	**8.5**	6	19.5	111	8.6	223	7.3	221	8.6	136	11.2
	I-V	**654**	**8.3**	6	20.9	102	8.4	202	6.9	214	8.5	130	11.0
	I	**37**	**6.4**	-	..	-	-	7	5.0	18	6.6	12	7.5
	II	**144**	**7.8**	-	-	12	10.6	45	8.2	53	7.2	34	7.5
	IIIN	**59**	**7.8**	-	-	6	7.8	13	4.5	26	9.2	14	13.2
	IIIM	**251**	**8.6**	2	16.9	43	8.7	83	6.9	74	8.5	49	15.2
	IV	**105**	**8.5**	1	16.7	23	6.8	34	6.7	33	11.6	14	13.9
	V	**58**	**10.**	3	37.8	18	9.5	20	8.9	10	12.8	7	17.6
	Others	**43**	**13.5**	-	-	9	11.9	21	13.4	7	12.0	6	23.5
3 and over	All	**544**	**12.2**	-	-	47	14.5	147	10.9	177	11.7	173	13.8
	I-V	**514**	**12.0**	-	-	45	14.4	134	10.4	169	11.7	166	13.6
	I	**30**	**12.2**	-	..	-	-	5	13.9	9	9.1	16	14.7
	II	**59**	**8.0**	-	..	2	8.4	12	8.5	24	8.8	21	6.9
	IIIN	**32**	**11.1**	-	..	-	-	12	15.9	15	13.5	5	5.4
	IIIM	**195**	**11.5**	-	-	18	12.8	56	10.0	58	9.9	63	15.5
	IV	**121**	**14.0**	-	-	15	16.5	26	8.4	41	15.7	39	19.1
	V	**77**	**17.5**	-	-	10	20.6	23	13.5	22	18.3	22	22.0
	Others	**30**	**17.9**	-	..	2	16.8	13	22.6	8	12.9	7	19.5
Illegitimate		**1,747**	**12.3**	**538**	**13.5**	**635**	**11.7**	**318**	**11.4**	**160**	**12.1**	**96**	**14.0**

Table 3 Neonatal deaths - numbers and rates per 1,000 live births: **England and Wales**
age of mother x parity, social class (legitimate only); 1986

Parity	Social class	Age of mother											
		All ages		Under 20		20 - 24		25 - 29		30 - 34		35 and over	
		Number	Rate	Number	Rate	Number	Rate	Number	Rate	Number	Rate	Number	Rate
All		**3,449**	**5.2**	**435**	**7.6**	**1,009**	**5.3**	**1,074**	**4.7**	**597**	**4.6**	**334**	**6.3**
All legitimate	All	**2,461**	**4.7**	103	5.8	645	4.7	917	4.6	519	4.5	277	6.0
	I-V	**2,289**	**4.6**	88	5.4	590	4.6	851	4.4	501	4.4	259	5.8
	I	**167**	**4.1**	1	4.3	12	3.0	67	4.2	55	3.8	32	5.3
	II	**485**	**4.1**	6	5.0	73	4.0	206	4.4	134	3.6	66	4.2
	IIIN	**237**	**4.3**	7	6.1	48	3.8	89	3.7	69	5.3	24	5.2
	IIIM	**841**	**4.7**	44	6.4	252	4.6	310	4.4	151	4.4	84	6.9
	IV	**391**	**5.4**	20	4.7	142	5.2	122	4.7	71	6.4	36	7.9
	V	**168**	**6.0**	10	3.9	63	5.3	57	6.4	21	6.6	17	9.8
	Others	**172**	**7.2**	15	10.4	55	6.1	66	7.7	18	5.1	18	14.8
0	All	**1,025**	**5.0**	82	5.9	340	4.6	380	4.8	166	5.4	57	6.9
	I-V	**946**	**4.8**	69	5.5	306	4.4	358	4.7	160	5.4	53	6.6
	I	**64**	**3.8**	-	-	9	3.5	31	3.6	19	4.2	5	4.1
	II	**208**	**4.3**	6	5.8	41	3.5	106	4.8	40	3.6	15	4.8
	IIIN	**102**	**4.2**	7	7.7	26	3.4	37	3.5	25	6.7	7	6.2
	IIIM	**361**	**5.3**	33	6.1	137	4.7	124	5.0	53	7.2	14	7.4
	IV	**159**	**5.8**	17	5.3	72	5.4	43	5.3	18	7.8	9	16.8
	V	**52**	**5.6**	6	3.2	21	4.4	17	8.7	5	10.2	3	20.5
	Others	**79**	**7.5**	13	10.6	34	6.8	22	7.2	6	6.2	4	15.8
1	All	**807**	**4.3**	18	4.9	210	4.4	335	4.3	170	3.8	74	5.5
	I-V	**753**	**4.2**	16	4.6	196	4.4	307	4.1	165	3.8	69	5.3
	I	**58**	**3.7**	1	14.0	3	2.3	27	4.6	18	2.9	9	4.3
	II	**168**	**3.8**	-	-	22	4.3	75	4.1	49	3.1	22	4.3
	IIIN	**95**	**4.6**	-	-	21	5.3	39	4.0	26	4.9	9	5.8
	IIIM	**269**	**4.1**	10	7.3	79	4.0	108	3.7	48	3.9	24	7.7
	IV	**121**	**4.9**	3	2.9	48	5.0	47	4.9	20	5.8	3	3.1
	V	**42**	**4.6**	2	3.4	23	4.9	11	3.7	4	5.5	2	9.6
	Others	**54**	**6.4**	2	9.8	14	4.4	28	8.3	5	3.7	5	14.1
2	All	**365**	**4.5**	3	9.9	69	5.3	117	3.8	104	4.0	72	6.0
	I-V	**347**	**4.4**	3	10.5	63	5.2	110	3.8	102	4.1	69	5.9
	I	**23**	**4.0**	-	..	-	-	4	2.9	11	4.0	8	5.0
	II	**81**	**4.4**	-	-	10	8.9	24	4.4	28	3.8	19	4.2
	IIIN	**25**	**3.3**	-	-	1	1.3	6	2.1	11	3.9	7	6.7
	IIIM	**127**	**4.4**	1	8.5	27	5.5	45	3.7	28	3.2	26	8.1
	IV	**60**	**4.9**	-	-	13	3.9	20	4.0	21	7.4	6	6.0
	V	**31**	**5.8**	2	25.5	12	6.4	11	4.9	3	3.9	3	7.6
	Others	**18**	**5.7**	-	-	6	7.9	7	4.5	2	3.5	3	11.9
3 and over	All	**264**	**6.0**	-	-	26	8.1	85	6.3	79	5.3	74	6.0
	I-V	**243**	**5.7**	-	-	25	8.1	76	5.9	74	5.1	68	5.6
	I	**22**	**9.0**	-	..	-	-	5	13.9	7	7.1	10	9.2
	II	**28**	**3.8**	-	..	-	-	1	0.7	17	6.3	10	3.3
	IIIN	**15**	**5.3**	-	..	-	-	7	9.3	7	6.4	1	1.1
	IIIM	**84**	**5.0**	-	-	9	6.5	33	5.9	22	3.8	20	5.0
	IV	**51**	**5.9**	-	-	9	10.0	12	3.9	12	4.7	18	8.9
	V	**43**	**9.9**	-	-	7	14.5	18	10.6	9	7.6	9	9.1
	Others	**21**	**12.6**	-	..	1	8.5	9	15.8	5	8.1	6	16.7
Illegitimate		**988**	**7.0**	332	8.4	364	6.7	157	5.7	78	5.9	57	8.4

Table 4 Postneonatal deaths - numbers and rates per 1,000 live births: age of mother x parity, social class (legitimate only); 1986

England and Wales

Parity	Social class	Age of mother											
		All ages		Under 20		20 - 24		25 - 29		30 - 34		35 and over	
		Number	Rate	Number	Rate	Number	Rate	Number	Rate	Number	Rate	Number	Rate
ALL		2,760	4.2	412	7.2	959	5.0	814	3.6	387	3.0	188	3.5
All legitimate	All	1,901	3.7	121	6.8	613	4.4	665	3.3	342	2.9	160	3.5
	I-V	1,737	3.5	100	6.1	549	4.3	617	3.2	316	2.8	155	3.4
	I	109	2.7	1	4.3	6	1.5	41	2.5	42	2.9	19	3.2
	II	353	3.0	8	6.7	54	3.0	142	3.0	103	2.8	46	2.9
	IIIN	168	3.0	6	5.2	53	4.2	68	2.8	30	2.3	11	2.4
	IIIM	616	3.4	33	4.8	237	4.3	202	2.8	95	2.8	49	4.0
	IV	344	4.7	27	6.3	139	5.1	122	4.7	31	2.8	25	5.5
	V	147	5.2	25	9.8	60	5.1	42	4.7	15	4.7	5	2.9
	Others	164	6.9	21	14.5	64	7.1	48	5.6	26	7.4	5	4.1
0	All	538	2.6	77	5.6	200	2.7	183	2.3	60	2.0	18	2.2
	I-V	494	2.5	63	5.0	186	2.7	171	2.3	56	1.9	18	2.2
	I	32	1.9	1	6.2	1	0.4	17	2.0	11	2.5	2	1.6
	II	99	2.0	5	4.8	26	2.2	40	1.8	21	1.9	7	2.2
	IIIN	59	2.5	6	6.6	22	2.9	22	2.1	7	1.9	2	1.8
	IIIM	172	2.5	19	3.5	79	2.7	59	2.4	12	1.6	3	1.6
	IV	93	3.4	17	5.3	41	3.1	28	3.5	3	1.3	4	7.5
	V	39	4.2	15	8.0	17	3.6	5	2.6	2	4.1	-	-
	Others	44	4.2	14	11.4	14	2.8	12	3.9	4	4.1	-	-
1	All	725	3.8	43	11.7	265	5.6	243	3.1	125	2.8	49	3.6
	I-V	661	3.7	36	10.4	231	5.2	229	3.0	118	2.7	47	3.6
	I	55	3.5	-	-	3	2.3	21	3.6	23	3.7	8	3.8
	II	143	3.2	3	21.0	19	3.7	62	3.4	47	3.0	12	2.3
	IIIN	57	2.7	-	-	18	4.6	26	2.7	9	1.7	4	2.6
	IIIM	229	3.5	14	10.2	110	5.6	63	2.2	28	2.3	14	4.5
	IV	130	5.3	10	9.6	59	6.2	46	4.8	8	2.3	7	7.2
	V	47	5.1	9	15.2	22	4.7	11	3.7	3	4.1	2	9.6
	Others	64	7.6	7	34.3	34	10.7	14	4.2	7	5.2	2	5.6
2	All	405	5.0	1	3.3	111	8.6	164	5.4	85	3.3	44	3.7
	I-V	366	4.7	1	3.5	98	8.1	149	5.1	76	3.0	42	3.6
	I	16	2.8	-	..	2	21.5	2	1.4	5	1.8	7	4.4
	II	75	4.1	-	-	5	4.4	32	5.9	26	3.5	12	2.7
	IIIN	39	5.2	-	-	8	10.5	18	6.3	10	3.6	3	2.9
	IIIM	127	4.4	-	-	37	7.5	50	4.2	26	3.0	14	4.4
	IV	74	6.0	-	-	31	9.3	31	6.1	7	2.5	5	5.0
	V	35	6.5	1	12.7	15	8.0	16	7.2	2	2.6	1	2.5
	Others	39	12.3	-	-	13	17.2	15	9.7	9	15.5	2	7.9
3 and over	All	233	5.3	-	-	37	11.5	75	5.6	72	4.8	49	3.9
	I-V	216	5.1	-	-	34	11.0	68	5.3	66	4.6	48	4.0
	I	6	2.5	-	..	-	-	1	2.8	3	3.0	2	1.8
	II	36	4.9	-	..	4	16.9	8	5.7	9	3.3	15	4.9
	IIIN	13	4.6	-	..	5	61.2	2	2.7	4	3.6	2	2.2
	IIIM	88	5.2	-	-	11	7.9	30	5.4	29	5.0	18	4.5
	IV	47	5.5	-	-	8	8.9	17	5.5	13	5.0	9	4.5
	V	26	6.0	-	-	6	12.5	10	5.9	8	6.7	2	2.0
	Others	17	10.2	-	..	3	25.4	7	12.3	6	9.7	1	2.8
Illegitimate		859	6.1	291	7.3	346	6.4	149	5.4	45	3.4	28	4.1

Table 5 Infant deaths - numbers and rates per 1,000 live births:
age of mother x parity, social class (legitimate only); 1986

England and Wales

Parity	Social class	Age of mother											
		All ages		Under 20		20 - 24		25 - 29		30 - 34		35 and over	
		Number	Rate	Number	Rate	Number	Rate	Number	Rate	Number	Rate	Number	Rate
All		**6,209**	**9.4**	**847**	**14.8**	**1,968**	**10.2**	**1,888**	**8.2**	**984**	**7.6**	**522**	**9.8**
All legitimate	All	4,362	8.4	224	12.6	1,258	9.1	1,582	7.9	861	7.4	437	9.5
	I-V	4,026	8.1	188	11.5	1,139	8.8	1,468	7.6	817	7.2	414	9.2
	I	276	6.8	2	8.5	18	4.5	108	6.7	97	6.7	51	8.5
	II	838	7.0	14	11.7	127	7.0	348	7.4	237	6.4	112	7.1
	IIIN	405	7.3	13	11.3	101	8.1	157	6.6	99	7.6	35	7.5
	IIIM	1,457	8.1	77	11.1	489	8.9	512	7.2	246	7.2	133	10.9
	IV	735	10.1	47	10.9	281	10.3	244	9.5	102	9.2	61	13.5
	V	315	11.2	35	13.7	123	10.4	99	11.2	36	11.3	22	12.7
	Others	336	14.1	36	24.9	119	13.1	114	13.3	44	12.6	23	18.9
0	All	1,563	7.6	159	11.5	540	7.3	563	7.1	226	7.4	75	9.0
	I-V	1,440	7.4	132	10.5	492	7.1	529	7.0	216	7.3	71	8.8
	I	96	5.6	1	6.2	10	3.9	48	5.6	30	6.7	7	5.7
	II	307	6.3	11	10.7	67	5.7	146	6.7	61	5.5	22	7.0
	IIIN	161	6.7	13	14.3	48	6.2	59	5.6	32	8.6	9	8.0
	IIIM	533	7.8	52	9.6	216	7.4	183	7.4	65	8.8	17	9.0
	IV	252	9.2	34	10.7	113	8.4	71	8.8	21	9.1	13	24.3
	V	91	9.9	21	11.2	38	8.0	22	11.3	7	14.3	3	20.5
	Others	123	11.7	27	22.1	48	9.6	34	11.1	10	10.3	4	15.8
1	All	1,532	8.1	61	16.6	475	10.0	578	7.4	295	6.5	123	9.1
	I-V	1,414	7.9	52	15.0	427	9.6	536	7.1	283	6.5	116	8.8
	I	113	7.3	1	14.0	6	4.7	48	8.2	41	6.5	17	8.1
	II	311	7.0	3	21.0	41	8.0	137	7.5	96	6.0	34	6.6
	IIIN	152	7.3	-	-	39	9.9	65	6.7	35	6.5	13	8.3
	IIIM	498	7.6	24	17.4	189	9.5	171	5.9	76	6.2	38	12.2
	IV	251	10.2	13	12.5	107	11.2	93	9.7	28	8.2	10	10.2
	V	89	9.6	11	18.6	45	9.5	22	7.4	7	9.6	4	19.3
	Others	118	14.0	9	44.1	48	15.1	42	12.5	12	9.0	7	19.7
2	All	770	9.5	4	13.2	180	13.9	281	9.2	189	7.4	116	9.7
	I-V	713	9.1	4	14.1	161	13.2	259	8.9	178	7.1	111	9.4
	I	39	6.7	-	..	2	21.5	6	4.3	16	5.9	15	9.4
	II	156	8.4	-	-	15	13.3	56	10.3	54	7.3	31	6.9
	IIIN	64	8.5	-	-	9	11.8	24	8.4	21	7.5	10	9.5
	IIIM	254	8.8	1	8.5	64	13.0	95	7.9	54	6.3	40	12.5
	IV	134	10.9	-	-	44	13.1	51	10.1	28	9.9	11	11.0
	V	66	12.3	3	38.2	27	14.3	27	12.1	5	6.5	4	10.2
	Others	57	18.0	-	-	19	25.2	22	14.2	11	19.0	5	19.8
3 and over	All	497	11.3	-	-	63	19.6	160	11.9	151	10.1	123	9.9
	I-V	459	10.8	-	-	59	19.0	144	11.2	140	9.7	116	9.6
	I	28	11.5	-	..	-	-	6	16.7	10	10.1	12	11.1
	II	64	8.7	-	..	4	16.9	9	6.5	26	9.6	25	8.2
	IIIN	28	9.8	-	..	5	61.2	9	12.0	11	10.0	3	3.2
	IIIM	172	10.2	-	-	20	14.4	63	11.3	51	8.8	38	9.5
	IV	98	11.4	-	-	17	18.9	29	9.4	25	9.7	27	13.4
	V	69	15.8	-	-	13	27.0	28	16.5	17	14.3	11	11.2
	Others	38	22.8	-	..	4	33.9	16	28.1	11	17.8	7	19.5
Illegitimate		**1,847**	**13.1**	**623**	**15.7**	**710**	**13.1**	**306**	**11.0**	**123**	**9.4**	**85**	**12.5**

Table 6 Live births - numbers (thousands): England and Wales
age of mother x parity, social class (legitimate only); 1986

Parity	Social class	Age of mother					
		All ages	Under 20	20 - 24	25 - 29	30 - 34	35 and over
All legitimate	All	519.7	17.8	138.0	201.3	116.4	46.2
	I-V	495.9	16.3	128.9	192.8	112.9	45.0
	I	40.8	0.2	4.0	16.1	14.5	6.0
	II	119.3	1.2	18.2	47.0	37.1	15.8
	IIIN	55.2	1.2	12.5	23.9	13.0	4.7
	IIIM	179.5	6.9	55.2	71.1	34.0	12.2
	IV	72.9	4.3	27.2	25.7	11.1	4.5
	V	28.2	2.6	11.9	8.9	3.2	1.7
	Others	23.8	1.4	9.1	8.6	3.5	1.2
0	All	205.6	13.8	74.3	78.8	30.5	8.3
	I-V	195.1	12.6	69.2	75.7	29.5	8.0
	I	17.0	0.2	2.6	8.5	4.5	1.2
	II	48.9	1.0	11.7	21.9	11.1	3.1
	IIIN	24.1	0.9	7.7	10.6	3.7	1.1
	IIIM	68.4	5.4	29.1	24.6	7.4	1.9
	IV	27.5	3.2	13.4	8.1	2.3	0.5
	V	9.2	1.9	4.8	1.9	0.5	0.1
	Others	10.5	1.2	5.0	3.1	1.0	0.3
1	All	188.5	3.7	47.6	78.6	45.2	13.5
	I-V	180.1	3.5	44.4	75.2	43.9	13.1
	I	15.6	0.1	1.3	5.8	6.3	2.1
	II	44.5	0.1	5.1	18.2	15.9	5.1
	IIIN	20.8	0.2	3.9	9.7	5.4	1.6
	IIIM	65.4	1.4	19.8	28.9	12.2	3.1
	IV	24.6	1.0	9.6	9.5	3.4	1.0
	V	9.2	0.6	4.7	3.0	0.7	0.2
	Others	8.4	0.2	3.2	3.4	1.3	0.4
2	All	81.5	0.3	12.9	30.6	25.7	12.0
	I-V	78.3	0.3	12.2	29.0	25.1	11.8
	I	5.8	-	0.1	1.4	2.7	1.6
	II	18.5	0.0	1.1	5.5	7.4	4.5
	IIIN	7.5	0.0	0.8	2.9	2.8	1.1
	IIIM	28.9	0.1	4.9	12.0	8.6	3.2
	IV	12.3	0.1	3.4	5.0	2.8	1.0
	V	5.4	0.1	1.9	2.2	0.8	0.4
	Others	3.2	0.0	0.8	1.6	0.6	0.3
3 and over	All	44.1	0.0	3.2	13.4	15.0	12.4
	I-V	42.4	0.0	3.1	12.9	14.4	12.1
	I	2.4	-	0.0	0.4	1.0	1.1
	II	7.4	-	0.2	1.4	2.7	3.0
	IIIN	2.9	-	0.1	0.7	1.1	0.9
	IIIM	16.8	0.0	1.4	5.6	5.8	4.0
	IV	8.6	0.0	0.9	3.1	2.6	2.0
	V	4.4	0.0	0.5	1.7	1.2	1.0
	Others	1.7	-	0.1	0.6	0.6	0.4
Live births	Legitimate	519,673	17,793	137,985	201,323	116,369	46,203
	Illegitimate	141,345	39,613	54,079	27,712	13,118	6,823

Table 7a Stillbirths, infant deaths and live births - numbers and rates per 1,000 total/live births†: age of infant x area of residence, social class (legitimate only); 1986

England and Wales, Wales and regional health authorities

Regional health authority of residence	Social class	Stillbirths		Perinatal deaths		Neonatal deaths		Postneonatal deaths		Infant deaths		Live births
		Number	Rate	Number	Rate	Number	Rate	Number	Rate	Number	Rate	Number
England and Wales *	All	2,600	5.0	4,591	8.8	2,461	4.7	1,901	3.7	4,362	8.4	519,673
	I-V	2,439	4.9	4,286	8.6	2,289	4.6	1,737	3.5	4,026	8.1	495,880
	I	150	3.7	293	7.2	167	4.1	109	2.7	276	6.8	40,810
	II	478	4.0	865	7.2	485	4.1	353	3.0	838	7.0	119,300
	III(N)	267	4.8	465	8.4	237	4.3	168	3.0	405	7.3	55,220
	III(M)	939	5.2	1,611	8.9	841	4.7	616	3.4	1,457	8.1	179,500
	IV	419	5.7	729	9.9	391	5.4	344	4.7	735	10.1	72,890
	V	186	6.6	323	11.4	168	6.0	147	5.2	315	11.2	28,170
Wales	All	154	5.2	287	9.8	158	5.4	111	3.8	269	9.2	29,215
	I-V	143	5.1	265	9.5	146	5.2	100	3.6	246	8.8	27,870
	I	5	2.9	13	7.4	11	6.3	2	1.1	13	7.4	1,750
	II	27	4.9	51	9.3	31	5.7	16	2.9	47	8.6	5,480
	III(N)	15	5.1	24	8.2	11	3.8	9	3.1	20	6.9	2,920
	III(M)	58	5.5	99	9.4	46	4.4	46	4.4	92	8.8	10,450
	IV	23	5.3	54	12.5	35	8.1	16	3.7	51	11.8	4,310
	V	15	5.0	24	8.0	12	4.0	11	3.7	23	7.7	2,970
Northern	All	157	5.1	301	9.8	170	5.6	100	3.3	270	8.9	30,430
	I-V	151	5.1	290	9.8	165	5.6	95	3.2	260	8.8	29,430
	I	4	2.1	13	7.0	11	5.9	4	2.1	15	8.1	1,860
	II	26	4.7	57	10.4	35	6.4	15	2.7	50	9.2	5,460
	III(N)	17	5.9	35	12.2	18	6.3	15	5.3	33	11.6	2,850
	III(M)	67	5.6	109	9.1	55	4.6	34	2.8	89	7.5	11,940
	IV	21	4.6	47	10.2	31	6.8	16	3.5	47	10.2	4,590
	V	16	5.8	29	10.5	15	5.5	11	4.0	26	9.5	2,740
Yorkshire	All	188	5.0	338	9.0	186	5.0	135	3.6	321	8.6	37,230
	I-V	183	5.1	328	9.1	179	5.0	128	3.6	307	8.6	35,780
	I	10	4.5	15	6.8	6	2.7	5	2.3	11	5.0	2,200
	II	34	4.6	57	7.8	29	4.0	23	3.1	52	7.1	7,320
	III(N)	18	4.6	34	8.8	21	5.4	11	2.8	32	8.3	3,860
	III(M)	62	4.6	117	8.7	66	4.9	39	2.9	105	7.9	13,340
	IV	35	5.5	64	10.0	34	5.3	31	4.9	65	10.2	6,380
	V	24	8.8	41	15.1	23	8.5	19	7.1	42	15.6	2,690
Trent	All	240	5.2	440	9.5	246	5.3	156	3.4	402	8.7	46,099
	I-V	232	5.2	422	9.4	236	5.3	144	3.2	380	8.5	44,630
	I	6	2.0	16	5.4	11	3.7	6	2.0	17	5.7	2,960
	II	47	5.2	87	9.7	52	5.8	20	2.2	72	8.1	8,940
	III(N)	16	3.7	35	8.0	21	4.8	11	2.5	32	7.3	4,360
	III(M)	94	5.3	172	9.7	96	5.4	54	3.0	150	8.5	17,720
	IV	45	5.7	74	9.4	39	5.0	39	5.0	78	10.0	7,820
	V	24	8.4	38	13.3	17	6.0	14	4.9	31	10.9	2,830
East Anglian	All	81	3.9	141	6.8	77	3.7	73	3.6	150	7.3	20,556
	I-V	71	3.9	120	6.5	63	3.4	64	3.5	127	6.9	18,330
	I	8	5.6	14	9.7	9	6.3	4	2.8	13	9.1	1,430
	II	11	2.4	20	4.4	12	2.6	13	2.8	25	5.5	4,580
	III(N)	8	3.8	15	7.1	9	4.3	5	2.4	14	6.6	2,120
	III(M)	21	3.2	35	5.4	16	2.5	27	4.2	43	6.6	6,500
	IV	18	6.8	27	10.2	11	4.2	8	3.0	19	7.2	2,630
	V	5	4.6	9	8.3	6	5.6	7	6.5	13	12.0	1,080
North West Thames	All	183	4.6	324	8.2	180	4.6	134	3.4	314	7.9	39,504
	I-V	176	4.6	304	8.0	166	4.4	122	3.2	288	7.6	38,010
	I	22	4.9	33	7.4	13	2.9	10	2.2	23	5.1	4,470
	II	42	3.6	76	6.5	49	4.2	32	2.7	81	7.0	11,640
	III(N)	32	6.4	53	10.6	23	4.6	17	3.4	40	8.0	4,990
	III(M)	52	4.5	86	7.4	45	3.9	37	3.2	82	7.1	11,630
	IV	20	4.7	39	9.2	25	5.9	21	5.0	46	10.9	4,220
	V	8	7.4	17	15.8	11	10.3	5	4.7	16	14.9	1,070
North East Thames	All	197	4.7	356	8.5	201	4.8	149	3.6	350	8.4	41,476
	I-V	187	4.7	328	8.2	179	4.5	138	3.5	317	8.0	39,820
	I	21	6.4	31	9.5	12	3.7	6	1.8	18	5.5	3,250
	II	34	3.2	61	5.8	37	3.5	26	2.5	63	6.0	10,440
	III(N)	25	5.3	41	8.6	21	4.5	19	4.0	40	8.5	4,720
	III(M)	66	4.8	121	8.8	68	4.9	49	3.6	117	8.5	13,760
	IV	31	5.1	51	8.4	27	4.5	30	5.0	57	9.5	6,020
	V	10	6.1	23	14.0	14	8.6	8	4.9	22	13.5	1,630

* Including births and deaths to persons normally resident outside England and Wales.
† See Definitions, page 4.

Table 7a - *continued*

Regional health authority of residence	Social class	Stillbirths		Perinatal deaths		Neonatal deaths		Postneonatal deaths		Infant deaths		Live births
		Number	Rate	Number	Rate	Number	Rate	Number	Rate	Number	Rate	Number
South East Thames	All	176	4.9	276	7.7	137	3.9	132	3.7	269	7.6	35,548
	I-V	166	4.9	261	7.6	128	3.8	118	3.5	246	7.2	34,040
	I	13	4.3	20	6.6	9	3.0	8	2.7	17	5.7	3,000
	II	40	4.4	59	6.5	23	2.5	28	3.1	51	5.6	9,090
	III(N)	25	5.7	37	8.5	18	4.2	11	2.5	29	6.7	4,320
	III(M)	67	5.5	107	8.8	52	4.3	42	3.5	94	7.8	12,090
	IV	13	3.3	23	5.8	19	4.8	23	5.8	42	10.6	3,970
	V	8	5.1	15	9.5	7	4.5	6	3.8	13	8.3	1,570
South West Thames	All	141	4.6	238	7.7	125	4.1	121	4.0	246	8.0	30,569
	I-V	134	4.5	227	7.7	119	4.0	113	3.8	232	7.9	29,520
	I	16	3.8	30	7.1	14	3.3	14	3.3	28	6.6	4,230
	II	29	3.0	59	6.0	41	4.2	34	3.5	75	7.7	9,790
	III(N)	11	2.7	20	4.9	15	3.7	12	3.0	27	6.7	4,030
	III(M)	52	6.4	80	9.8	35	4.3	28	3.4	63	7.7	8,130
	IV	21	8.0	28	10.6	7	2.7	20	7.7	27	10.3	2,610
	V	5	6.9	10	13.7	7	9.7	5	6.9	12	16.6	720
Wessex	All	154	5.1	250	8.4	132	4.4	114	3.8	246	8.3	29,758
	I-V	132	5.0	215	8.1	117	4.4	97	3.7	214	8.1	26,430
	I	8	3.3	14	5.8	8	3.3	9	3.7	17	7.1	2,410
	II	24	3.4	45	6.4	27	3.8	24	3.4	51	7.2	7,050
	III(N)	13	4.7	20	7.2	10	3.6	8	2.9	18	6.5	2,760
	III(M)	56	5.8	89	9.2	45	4.7	37	3.8	82	8.5	9,630
	IV	23	6.5	36	10.2	21	6.0	15	4.3	36	10.3	3,510
	V	8	7.4	11	10.2	6	5.6	4	3.7	10	9.4	1,070
Oxford	All	123	4.4	239	8.5	134	4.8	95	3.4	229	8.2	27,845
	I-V	109	4.1	213	8.1	120	4.6	85	3.2	205	7.8	26,290
	I	11	3.6	22	7.2	14	4.6	5	1.6	19	6.3	3,030
	II	28	3.8	49	6.7	23	3.2	22	3.0	45	6.2	7,300
	III(N)	13	4.5	24	8.4	13	4.6	6	2.1	19	6.7	2,850
	III(M)	37	4.2	83	9.5	51	5.9	31	3.6	82	9.4	8,690
	IV	17	4.9	27	7.9	13	3.8	18	5.3	31	9.1	3,420
	V	3	3.0	8	7.9	6	5.9	3	3.0	9	8.9	1,010
South Western	All	153	4.9	276	8.8	140	4.5	135	4.3	275	8.8	31,295
	I-V	142	4.9	257	8.8	130	4.5	124	4.3	254	8.8	29,030
	I	7	3.0	19	8.1	12	5.1	14	6.0	26	11.1	2,340
	II	41	5.5	61	8.3	23	3.1	28	3.8	51	6.9	7,350
	III(N)	15	4.9	32	10.4	18	5.9	12	3.9	30	9.8	3,050
	III(M)	47	4.4	89	8.3	51	4.8	44	4.1	95	8.9	10,670
	IV	24	5.6	41	9.6	19	4.5	18	4.3	37	8.7	4,230
	V	8	5.7	15	10.7	7	5.0	8	5.7	15	10.8	1,390
West Midlands	All	311	5.6	537	9.7	266	4.8	184	3.3	450	8.2	55,022
	I-V	290	5.4	506	9.4	254	4.8	171	3.2	425	8.0	53,400
	I	9	2.5	21	5.9	15	4.2	9	2.5	24	6.8	3,540
	II	42	3.7	93	8.1	58	5.1	28	2.4	86	7.5	11,440
	III(N)	20	3.8	34	6.5	16	3.1	14	2.7	30	5.7	5,220
	III(M)	129	6.0	210	9.8	97	4.5	60	2.8	157	7.3	21,370
	IV	72	8.0	122	13.5	60	6.7	42	4.8	102	11.5	8,970
	V	18	6.3	26	9.0	8	2.8	18	6.3	26	9.1	2,860
Mersey	All	120	5.0	208	8.6	113	4.7	93	3.9	206	8.6	24,024
	I-V	113	4.8	197	8.4	108	4.6	83	3.5	191	8.1	23,440
	I	4	2.3	10	5.9	6	3.5	6	3.5	12	7.1	1,700
	II	18	3.7	34	6.9	20	4.1	18	3.7	38	7.7	4,910
	III(N)	11	4.1	24	8.9	13	4.8	6	2.2	19	7.1	2,690
	III(M)	47	5.6	79	9.4	47	5.6	25	3.0	72	8.6	8,390
	IV	22	5.7	32	8.3	14	3.6	19	5.0	33	8.6	3,840
	V	11	5.7	18	9.4	8	4.2	9	4.7	17	8.9	1,900
North Western	All	219	5.3	374	9.1	193	4.7	169	4.1	362	8.9	40,776
	I-V	207	5.2	347	8.7	176	4.4	155	3.9	331	8.3	39,650
	I	6	2.3	22	8.4	16	6.1	7	2.7	23	8.8	2,610
	II	34	4.0	54	6.3	24	2.8	26	3.1	50	5.9	8,480
	III(N)	27	6.0	35	7.8	9	2.0	12	2.7	21	4.7	4,440
	III(M)	83	5.4	133	8.7	70	4.6	63	4.2	133	8.8	15,170
	IV	34	5.4	64	10.2	36	5.7	28	4.5	64	10.2	6,270
	V	23	8.5	39	14.4	21	7.8	19	7.1	40	14.9	2,690

13

Table 7b   Stillbirths, infant deaths and live births - numbers and rates per 1,000 total/live births†: age of infant x area of residence, age of mother; 1986

England and Wales, Wales and regional health authorities

Regional health authority of residence	Age of mother	Stillbirths		Perinatal deaths		Neonatal deaths		Postneonatal deaths		Infant deaths		Live births
		Number	Rate	Number	Rate	Number	Rate	Number	Rate	Number	Rate	Number
England and Wales *	All ages	3,549	5.3	6,338	9.5	3,449	5.2	2,760	4.2	6,209	9.4	661,018
	Under 20	367	6.4	728	12.6	435	7.6	412	7.2	847	14.8	57,406
	20-24	1,017	5.3	1,823	9.4	1,009	5.3	959	5.0	1,968	10.2	192,064
	25-29	1,098	4.8	1,948	8.5	1,074	4.7	814	3.6	1,888	8.2	229,035
	30-34	680	5.2	1,172	9.0	597	4.6	387	3.0	984	7.6	129,487
	35 and over	387	7.2	667	12.5	334	6.3	188	3.5	522	9.8	53,026
Wales	All ages	209	5.6	384	10.3	207	5.6	143	3.9	350	9.4	37,038
	Under 20	32	8.2	47	12.1	19	4.9	22	5.7	41	10.6	3,855
	20-24	46	3.8	97	8.1	60	5.0	50	4.2	110	9.2	11,984
	25-29	71	5.7	125	10.1	68	5.5	49	4.0	117	9.5	12,314
	30-34	40	6.3	71	11.1	34	5.4	17	2.7	51	8.1	6,331
	35 and over	20	7.8	44	17.1	26	10.2	5	2.0	31	12.1	2,554
Northern	All ages	223	5.5	409	10.1	235	5.8	154	3.8	389	9.7	40,239
	Under 20	32	7.0	53	11.5	29	6.4	31	6.8	60	13.2	4,559
	20-24	72	5.6	129	10.0	72	5.6	47	3.7	119	9.3	12,842
	25-29	56	4.1	124	9.1	83	6.1	52	3.8	135	9.9	13,598
	30-34	41	6.0	66	9.6	30	4.4	18	2.6	48	7.0	6,829
	35 and over	22	9.0	37	15.2	21	8.7	6	2.5	27	11.2	2,411
Yorkshire	All ages	261	5.4	499	10.3	290	6.0	222	4.6	512	10.6	48,340
	Under 20	30	5.8	81	15.8	60	11.8	41	8.0	101	19.8	5,104
	20-24	80	5.2	137	8.9	76	5.0	95	6.2	171	11.2	15,264
	25-29	82	5.0	161	9.8	96	5.8	60	3.7	156	9.5	16,419
	30-34	44	5.2	74	8.7	35	4.1	13	1.5	48	5.7	8,450
	35 and over	25	8.0	46	14.7	23	7.4	13	4.2	36	11.6	3,103
Trent	All ages	324	5.4	603	10.1	349	5.9	234	3.9	583	9.8	59,284
	Under 20	39	6.6	75	12.6	43	7.3	47	7.9	90	15.2	5,914
	20-24	92	4.9	186	9.9	121	6.5	98	5.3	219	11.7	18,661
	25-29	103	5.0	183	8.9	104	5.1	57	2.8	161	7.9	20,407
	30-34	50	4.8	88	8.4	49	4.7	22	2.1	71	6.8	10,406
	35 and over	40	10.2	71	18.0	32	8.2	10	2.6	42	10.8	3,896
East Anglian	All ages	111	4.5	190	7.7	101	4.1	96	3.9	197	8.0	24,592
	Under 20	10	5.5	17	9.4	9	5.0	10	5.6	19	10.6	1,797
	20-24	32	4.3	51	6.9	29	3.9	32	4.4	61	8.3	7,343
	25-29	30	3.4	63	7.1	38	4.3	37	4.2	75	8.5	8,809
	30-34	23	4.8	36	7.5	16	3.4	12	2.5	28	5.9	4,772
	35 and over	16	8.5	23	12.2	9	4.8	5	2.7	14	7.5	1,871
North West Thames	All ages	230	4.8	414	8.6	232	4.8	179	3.7	411	8.5	48,124
	Under 20	11	4.1	26	9.7	16	6.0	18	6.7	34	12.7	2,682
	20-24	48	4.2	96	8.3	64	5.6	53	4.6	117	10.2	11,484
	25-29	95	5.5	160	9.2	81	4.7	65	3.8	146	8.4	17,325
	30-34	52	4.5	86	7.4	47	4.1	28	2.4	75	6.5	11,527
	35 and over	24	4.7	46	9.0	24	4.7	15	2.9	39	7.6	5,106
North East Thames	All ages	283	5.3	507	9.5	280	5.3	202	3.8	482	9.1	52,959
	Under 20	20	5.3	51	13.5	32	8.5	19	5.0	51	13.5	3,765
	20-24	86	5.9	139	9.6	68	4.7	63	4.4	131	9.1	14,433
	25-29	77	4.1	147	7.9	95	5.1	67	3.6	162	8.7	18,616
	30-34	63	5.6	106	9.4	49	4.4	30	2.7	79	7.1	11,172
	35 and over	37	7.4	64	12.8	36	7.2	23	4.6	59	11.9	4,973
South East Thames	All ages	261	5.5	407	8.5	195	4.1	209	4.4	404	8.5	47,558
	Under 20	27	7.4	40	10.9	16	4.4	40	11.0	56	15.4	3,632
	20-24	78	5.8	116	8.6	54	4.0	70	5.2	124	9.2	13,470
	25-29	77	4.6	123	7.3	63	3.8	53	3.2	116	6.9	16,723
	30-34	48	4.9	76	7.8	36	3.7	32	3.3	68	7.0	9,667
	35 and over	31	7.6	52	12.7	26	6.4	14	3.4	40	9.8	4,066
South West Thames	All ages	171	4.6	301	8.2	166	4.5	164	4.5	330	9.0	36,734
	Under 20	17	8.6	35	17.7	22	11.2	15	7.6	37	18.8	1,964
	20-24	38	4.8	69	8.7	36	4.6	43	5.5	79	10.1	7,856
	25-29	57	4.4	103	7.9	58	4.5	49	3.8	107	8.3	12,948
	30-34	34	3.5	55	5.7	32	3.3	39	4.1	71	7.4	9,564
	35 and over	25	5.6	39	8.8	18	4.1	18	4.1	36	8.2	4,402

* Including births and deaths to persons normally resident outside England and Wales.
† See Definitions, page 4.

Table 7b - *continued*

Regional health authority of residence	Age of mother	Stillbirths		Perinatal deaths		Neonatal deaths		Postneonatal deaths		Infant deaths		Live births
		Number	Rate	Number	Rate	Number	Rate	Number	Rate	Number	Rate	Number
Wessex	**All ages**	**187**	**5.2**	**316**	**8.8**	**171**	**4.8**	**144**	**4.0**	**315**	**8.8**	**35,772**
	Under 20	11	4.2	25	9.6	22	8.4	15	5.8	37	14.2	2,606
	20-24	66	6.4	106	10.2	47	4.6	49	4.7	96	9.3	10,322
	25-29	61	4.7	103	7.9	56	4.3	37	2.9	93	7.2	12,955
	30-34	32	4.5	51	7.2	29	4.1	29	4.1	58	8.2	7,095
	35 and over	17	6.0	31	11.0	17	6.1	14	5.0	31	11.1	2,794
Oxford	**All ages**	**147**	**4.4**	**294**	**8.8**	**173**	**5.2**	**116**	**3.5**	**289**	**8.7**	**33,201**
	Under 20	9	4.0	27	12.0	23	10.3	10	4.5	33	14.8	2,233
	20-24	31	3.6	61	7.1	34	4.0	44	5.1	78	9.1	8,600
	25-29	59	4.9	116	9.6	67	5.6	35	2.9	102	8.5	12,043
	30-34	30	4.0	60	8.1	34	4.6	21	2.8	55	7.4	7,413
	35 and over	18	6.1	30	10.2	15	5.2	6	2.1	21	7.2	2,912
South Western	**All ages**	**212**	**5.5**	**363**	**9.5**	**176**	**4.6**	**186**	**4.9**	**362**	**9.5**	**38,119**
	Under 20	15	5.3	26	9.3	14	5.0	24	8.6	38	13.6	2,789
	20-24	85	7.6	135	12.0	61	5.5	60	5.4	121	10.9	11,126
	25-29	50	3.6	98	7.1	54	3.9	62	4.5	116	8.4	13,764
	30-34	40	5.4	72	9.8	36	4.9	25	3.4	61	8.3	7,341
	35 and over	22	7.0	32	10.3	11	3.5	15	4.8	26	8.4	3,099
West Midlands	**All ages**	**425**	**6.0**	**771**	**10.9**	**406**	**5.8**	**287**	**4.1**	**693**	**9.8**	**70,408**
	Under 20	41	5.9	91	13.2	57	8.3	41	6.0	98	14.3	6,852
	20-24	128	5.9	247	11.5	140	6.5	111	5.2	251	11.7	21,436
	25-29	122	5.1	191	8.0	87	3.7	78	3.3	165	7.0	23,617
	30-34	88	6.7	166	12.6	87	6.6	36	2.8	123	9.4	13,090
	35 and over	46	8.4	76	13.9	35	6.5	21	3.9	56	10.3	5,413
Mersey	**All ages**	**180**	**5.5**	**299**	**9.1**	**157**	**4.8**	**146**	**4.5**	**303**	**9.3**	**32,712**
	Under 20	24	7.5	38	11.9	19	6.0	30	9.4	49	15.4	3,179
	20-24	48	4.9	85	8.7	49	5.0	38	3.9	87	9.0	9,715
	25-29	64	5.7	96	8.6	44	4.0	38	3.4	82	7.4	11,110
	30-34	34	5.4	58	9.3	30	4.8	31	5.0	61	9.8	6,206
	35 and over	10	4.0	22	8.8	15	6.0	9	3.6	24	9.6	2,502
North Western	**All ages**	**322**	**5.8**	**575**	**10.3**	**308**	**5.5**	**278**	**5.0**	**586**	**10.5**	**55,567**
	Under 20	49	7.5	96	14.8	54	8.4	49	7.6	103	16.0	6,456
	20-24	87	5.0	169	9.6	98	5.6	106	6.1	204	11.7	17,429
	25-29	92	5.0	153	8.3	80	4.4	75	4.1	155	8.5	18,272
	30-34	60	6.3	103	10.7	50	5.2	34	3.6	84	8.8	9,531
	35 and over	34	8.7	54	13.8	26	6.7	14	3.6	40	10.3	3,879

**Table 7c   Stillbirths, infant deaths and live births - numbers and rates
per 1,000 total/live births†: age of infant x area of
residence, parity (legitimate only); 1986**

England and Wales, Wales
and regional health authorities

Regional health authority of residence	Parity	Stillbirths		Perinatal deaths		Neonatal deaths		Postneonatal deaths		Infant deaths		Live births
		Number	Rate	Number	Rate	Number	Rate	Number	Rate	Number	Rate	Number
England and Wales *	All	3,549	5.3	6,338	9.5	3,449	5.2	2,760	4.2	6,209	9.4	661,018
	All Legitimate	2,600	5.0	4,591	8.8	2,461	4.7	1,901	3.7	4,362	8.4	519,673
	0	1,141	5.5	1,971	9.5	1,025	5.0	538	2.6	1,563	7.6	205,586
	1	731	3.9	1,379	7.3	807	4.3	725	3.8	1,532	8.1	188,539
	2	403	4.9	697	8.5	365	4.5	405	5.0	770	9.5	81,460
	3 and over	325	7.3	544	12.2	264	6.0	233	5.3	497	11.3	44,088
	Illegitimate	949	6.7	1,747	12.3	988	7.0	859	6.1	1,847	13.1	141,345
Wales	All	209	5.6	384	10.3	207	5.6	143	3.9	350	9.4	37,038
	All Legitimate	154	5.2	287	9.8	158	5.4	111	3.8	269	9.2	29,215
	0	63	5.5	122	10.6	73	6.4	36	3.2	109	9.5	11,421
	1	48	4.5	90	8.4	44	4.1	37	3.5	81	7.6	10,683
	2	27	5.6	47	9.7	26	5.4	27	5.6	53	11.0	4,814
	3 and over	16	6.9	28	12.1	15	6.5	11	4.8	26	11.3	2,297
	Illegitimate	55	7.0	97	12.3	49	6.3	32	4.1	81	10.4	7,823
Northern	All	223	5.5	409	10.1	235	5.8	154	3.8	389	9.7	40,239
	All Legitimate	157	5.1	301	9.8	170	5.6	100	3.3	270	8.9	30,430
	0	73	6.0	138	11.4	73	6.1	29	2.4	102	8.5	12,003
	1	49	4.2	93	8.0	58	5.0	38	3.3	96	8.3	11,567
	2	23	4.9	39	8.3	18	3.8	22	4.7	40	8.6	4,678
	3 and over	12	5.5	31	14.1	21	9.6	11	5.0	32	14.7	2,182
	Illegitimate	66	6.7	108	10.9	65	6.6	54	5.5	119	12.1	9,809
Yorkshire	All	261	5.4	499	10.3	290	6.0	222	4.6	512	10.6	48,340
	All Legitimate	188	5.0	338	9.0	186	5.0	135	3.6	321	8.6	37,230
	0	80	5.4	142	9.6	73	5.0	43	2.9	116	7.9	14,645
	1	54	4.1	101	7.6	66	5.0	48	3.6	114	8.6	13,202
	2	29	5.1	54	9.5	28	4.9	25	4.4	53	9.4	5,665
	3 and over	25	6.7	41	11.0	19	5.1	19	5.1	38	10.2	3,718
	Illegitimate	73	6.5	161	14.4	104	9.4	87	7.8	191	17.2	11,110
Trent	All	324	5.4	603	10.1	349	5.9	234	3.9	583	9.8	59,284
	All Legitimate	240	5.2	440	9.5	246	5.3	156	3.4	402	8.7	46,099
	0	103	5.5	202	10.8	122	6.6	46	2.5	168	9.1	18,552
	1	68	4.0	126	7.3	73	4.3	58	3.4	131	7.6	17,147
	2	40	5.7	63	9.0	27	3.9	34	4.9	61	8.8	6,923
	3 and over	29	8.3	49	14.0	24	6.9	18	5.2	42	12.1	3,477
	Illegitimate	84	6.3	163	12.3	103	7.8	78	5.9	181	13.7	13,185
East Anglian	All	111	4.5	190	7.7	101	4.1	96	3.9	197	8.0	24,592
	All Legitimate	81	3.9	141	6.8	77	3.7	73	3.6	150	7.3	20,556
	0	32	3.8	60	7.2	35	4.2	16	1.9	51	6.1	8,342
	1	31	4.0	54	7.0	31	4.0	35	4.5	66	8.6	7,694
	2	14	4.5	19	6.2	7	2.3	14	4.6	21	6.8	3,074
	3 and over	4	2.8	8	5.5	4	2.8	8	5.5	12	8.3	1,446
	Illegitimate	30	7.4	49	12.1	24	5.9	23	5.7	47	11.6	4,036
North West Thames	All	230	4.8	414	8.6	232	4.8	179	3.7	411	8.5	48,124
	All Legitimate	183	4.6	324	8.2	180	4.6	134	3.4	314	7.9	39,504
	0	94	5.8	149	9.2	71	4.4	37	2.3	108	6.7	16,154
	1	46	3.3	91	6.5	55	3.9	53	3.8	108	7.7	14,028
	2	20	3.3	40	6.5	28	4.6	24	3.9	52	8.5	6,106
	3 and over	23	7.1	44	13.6	26	8.1	20	6.2	46	14.3	3,216
	Illegitimate	47	5.4	90	10.4	52	6.0	45	5.2	97	11.3	8,620

* Including births and deaths to persons normally resident outside England and Wales.
† See Definitions, page 4.

Table 7c - *continued*

Regional health authority of residence	Parity	Stillbirths		Perinatal deaths		Neonatal deaths		Postneonatal deaths		Infant deaths		Live births
		Number	Rate	Number	Rate	Number	Rate	Number	Rate	Number	Rate	Number
North East Thames	**All**	**283**	**5.3**	**507**	**9.5**	**280**	**5.3**	**202**	**3.8**	**482**	**9.1**	**52,959**
	All Legitimate	197	4.7	356	8.5	201	4.8	149	3.6	350	8.4	41,476
	0	73	4.4	132	8.0	81	4.9	40	2.4	121	7.4	16,378
	1	56	3.9	118	8.1	70	4.9	54	3.7	124	8.6	14,425
	2	37	5.8	62	9.6	35	5.5	31	4.8	66	10.3	6,392
	3 and over	31	7.2	44	10.2	15	3.5	24	5.6	39	9.1	4,281
	Illegitimate	86	7.4	151	13.1	79	6.9	53	4.6	132	11.5	11,483
South East Thames	**All**	**261**	**5.5**	**407**	**8.5**	**195**	**4.1**	**209**	**4.4**	**404**	**8.5**	**47,558**
	All Legitimate	176	4.9	276	7.7	137	3.9	132	3.7	269	7.6	35,548
	0	81	5.6	109	7.5	44	3.1	43	3.0	87	6.1	14,368
	1	54	4.1	96	7.4	54	4.2	53	4.1	107	8.3	12,963
	2	26	4.7	44	8.0	22	4.0	25	4.6	47	8.6	5,494
	3 and over	15	5.5	27	9.9	17	6.2	11	4.0	28	10.3	2,723
	Illegitimate	85	7.0	131	10.8	58	4.8	77	6.4	135	11.2	12,010
South West Thames	**All**	**171**	**4.6**	**301**	**8.2**	**166**	**4.5**	**164**	**4.5**	**330**	**9.0**	**36,734**
	All Legitimate	141	4.6	238	7.7	125	4.1	121	4.0	246	8.0	30,569
	0	68	5.3	111	8.7	53	4.2	40	3.2	93	7.3	12,680
	1	41	3.6	69	6.1	36	3.2	43	3.8	79	7.0	11,312
	2	21	4.4	38	8.0	25	5.3	28	5.9	53	11.2	4,724
	3 and over	11	5.9	20	10.7	11	5.9	10	5.4	21	11.3	1,853
	Illegitimate	30	4.8	63	10.2	41	6.7	43	7.0	84	13.6	6,165
Wessex	**All**	**187**	**5.2**	**316**	**8.8**	**171**	**4.8**	**144**	**4.0**	**315**	**8.8**	**35,772**
	All Legitimate	154	5.1	250	8.4	132	4.4	114	3.8	246	8.3	29,758
	0	71	5.8	112	9.2	57	4.7	24	2.0	81	6.7	12,108
	1	51	4.5	82	7.3	43	3.8	50	4.5	93	8.3	11,194
	2	22	4.8	33	7.2	17	3.7	27	5.9	44	9.7	4,558
	3 and over	10	5.2	23	12.1	15	7.9	13	6.8	28	14.8	1,898
	Illegitimate	33	5.5	66	10.9	39	6.5	30	5.0	69	11.5	6,014
Oxford	**All**	**147**	**4.4**	**294**	**8.8**	**173**	**5.2**	**116**	**3.5**	**289**	**8.7**	**33,201**
	All Legitimate	123	4.4	239	8.5	134	4.8	95	3.4	229	8.2	27,845
	0	64	5.8	117	10.7	58	5.3	30	2.7	88	8.1	10,915
	1	30	2.9	72	6.9	51	4.9	35	3.4	86	8.3	10,362
	2	15	3.4	30	6.8	16	3.7	20	4.6	36	8.2	4,383
	3 and over	14	6.4	20	9.1	9	4.1	10	4.6	19	8.7	2,185
	Illegitimate	24	4.5	55	10.2	39	7.3	21	3.9	60	11.2	5,356
South Western	**All**	**212**	**5.5**	**363**	**9.5**	**176**	**4.6**	**186**	**4.9**	**362**	**9.5**	**38,119**
	All Legitimate	153	4.9	276	8.8	140	4.5	135	4.3	275	8.8	31,295
	0	70	5.5	127	10.0	65	5.1	37	2.9	102	8.1	12,644
	1	45	3.9	86	7.4	46	4.0	58	5.0	104	8.9	11,626
	2	22	4.5	42	8.6	23	4.7	27	5.6	50	10.3	4,851
	3 and over	16	7.3	21	9.6	6	2.8	13	6.0	19	8.7	2,174
	Illegitimate	59	8.6	87	12.6	36	5.3	51	7.5	87	12.7	6,824
West Midlands	**All**	**425**	**6.0**	**771**	**10.9**	**406**	**5.8**	**287**	**4.1**	**693**	**9.8**	**70,408**
	All Legitimate	311	5.6	537	9.7	266	4.8	184	3.3	450	8.2	55,022
	0	131	6.2	221	10.5	108	5.1	43	2.0	151	7.2	20,986
	1	65	3.4	129	6.7	75	3.9	74	3.8	149	7.7	19,260
	2	52	5.9	92	10.4	44	5.0	38	4.3	82	9.3	8,806
	3 and over	63	10.4	95	15.7	39	6.5	29	4.9	68	11.4	5,970
	Illegitimate	114	7.4	234	15.1	140	9.1	103	6.7	243	15.8	15,386

Table 7c - *continued*

Regional health authority of residence	Parity	Stillbirths		Perinatal deaths		Neonatal deaths		Postneonatal deaths		Infant deaths		Live births
		Number	Rate	Number	Rate	Number	Rate	Number	Rate	Number	Rate	Number
Mersey	**All**	**180**	**5.5**	**299**	**9.1**	**157**	**4.8**	**146**	**4.5**	**303**	**9.3**	**32,712**
	All Legitimate	120	5.0	208	8.6	113	4.7	93	3.9	206	8.6	24,024
	0	54	6.0	88	9.8	41	4.6	27	3.0	68	7.6	8,901
	1	32	3.6	62	7.1	40	4.6	29	3.3	69	7.9	8,756
	2	14	*3.3*	26	6.0	18	*4.2*	24	5.6	42	9.8	4,293
	3 and over	20	9.6	32	15.3	14	*6.8*	13	*6.3*	27	13.0	2,074
	Illegitimate	60	6.9	91	10.4	44	5.1	53	6.1	97	11.2	8,688
North Western	**All**	**322**	**5.8**	**575**	**10.3**	**308**	**5.5**	**278**	**5.0**	**586**	**10.5**	**55,567**
	All Legitimate	219	5.3	374	9.1	193	4.7	169	4.1	362	8.9	40,776
	0	83	5.4	140	9.1	71	4.6	47	3.1	118	7.7	15,345
	1	60	4.2	107	7.5	63	4.4	60	4.2	123	8.7	14,209
	2	40	6.0	66	9.9	30	4.5	39	5.9	69	10.4	6,652
	3 and over	36	7.8	61	13.2	29	6.3	23	5.0	52	11.4	4,570
	Illegitimate	103	6.9	201	13.5	115	7.8	109	7.4	224	15.1	14,791

Table 7d Stillbirths, infant deaths and live births: numbers and rates per 1,000 total/live births†: age by area of residence, birthweight, 1986

England and Wales

Regional health authority of residence	Birthweight (grams)	Stillbirths		Perinatal deaths		Neonatal deaths		Postneonatal deaths		Infant deaths		Live births
		Number	Rate	Number	Rate	Number	Rate	Number	Rate	Number	Rate	Number
England and Wales *	**All weights**	**3,549**	**5.3**	**6,338**	**9.5**	**3,449**	**5.2**	**2,760**	**4.2**	**6,209**	**9.4**	**661,018**
	Under 2,500	2,208	46.1	4,141	86.4	2,282	49.9	706	15.4	2,988	65.3	45,728
	Under 1,500	1,118	155.3	2,487	345.5	1,595	262.3	244	40.1	1,839	302.4	6,081
	1,500-1,999	501	53.3	799	85.0	357	40.1	186	20.9	543	61.1	8,894
	2,000-2,499	589	18.8	855	27.3	330	10.7	276	9.0	606	19.7	30,753
	2,500-2,999	529	4.4	798	6.6	365	3.0	591	4.9	956	8.0	119,810
	3,000-3,499	466	1.8	748	3.0	403	1.6	816	3.2	1,219	4.8	252,035
	3,500 and over	318	1.3	529	2.2	297	1.2	636	2.6	933	3.8	242,821
	Not stated	28	42.9	122	187.1	102	163.5	11	17.6	113	181.1	624
Wales	**All weights**	**209**	**5.6**	**384**	**10.3**	**207**	**5.6**	**143**	**3.9**	**350**	**9.4**	**37,038**
	Under 2,500	123	47.7	234	90.7	127	51.7	35	14.2	162	65.9	2,457
	Under 1,500	59	156.1	133	351.9	86	269.6	16	50.2	102	319.7	319
	1,500-1,999	27	49.9	46	85.0	19	37.0	8	15.6	27	52.5	514
	2,000-2,499	37	22.3	55	33.1	22	13.5	11	6.8	33	20.3	1,624
	2,500-2,999	27	4.2	47	7.3	21	3.3	26	4.1	47	7.4	6,369
	3,000-3,499	35	2.5	53	3.8	25	1.8	41	2.9	66	4.7	13,928
	3,500 and over	21	1.5	38	2.7	25	1.8	39	2.7	64	4.5	14,257
	Not stated	3	100.0	12	400.0	9	333.3	2	74.1	11	407.4	27
Northern	**All weights**	**223**	**5.5**	**409**	**10.1**	**235**	**5.8**	**154**	**3.8**	**389**	**9.7**	**40,239**
	Under 2,500	139	48.2	264	91.6	150	54.7	43	15.7	193	70.3	2,744
	Under 1,500	80	180.6	174	392.8	108	297.5	14	38.6	122	336.1	363
	1,500-1,999	18	35.0	38	73.9	24	48.4	6	12.1	30	60.5	496
	2,000-2,499	41	21.3	52	27.0	18	9.5	23	12.2	41	21.8	1,885
	2,500-2,999	32	4.5	48	6.7	19	2.7	33	4.6	52	7.3	7,148
	3,000-3,499	34	2.2	57	3.7	37	2.4	43	2.8	80	5.2	15,282
	3,500 and over	18	1.2	36	2.4	23	1.5	33	2.2	56	3.7	15,037
	Not stated	-	-	4	142.9	6	214.3	2	71.4	8	285.7	28
Yorkshire	**All weights**	**261**	**5.4**	**499**	**10.3**	**290**	**6.0**	**222**	**4.6**	**512**	**10.6**	**48,340**
	Under 2,500	164	44.2	327	88.0	187	52.7	57	16.1	244	68.7	3,550
	Under 1,500	78	149.4	199	381.2	134	301.8	14	31.5	148	333.3	444
	1,500-1,999	43	57.9	66	88.8	27	38.6	20	28.6	47	67.1	700
	2,000-2,499	43	17.6	62	25.3	26	10.8	23	9.6	49	20.4	2,406
	2,500-2,999	43	4.6	71	7.6	36	3.9	53	5.7	89	9.6	9,245
	3,000-3,499	31	1.7	54	2.9	35	1.9	59	3.2	94	5.1	18,573
	3,500 and over	20	1.2	38	2.2	25	1.5	52	3.1	77	4.5	16,956
	Not stated	3	157.9	9	473.7	7	437.5	1	62.5	8	500.0	16
Trent	**All weights**	**324**	**5.4**	**603**	**10.1**	**349**	**5.9**	**234**	**3.9**	**583**	**9.8**	**59,284**
	Under 2,500	202	44.9	399	88.6	239	55.6	60	14.0	299	69.5	4,300
	Under 1,500	104	148.6	248	354.3	168	281.9	22	36.9	190	318.8	596
	1,500-1,999	46	54.0	69	81.0	29	36.0	12	14.9	41	50.9	806
	2,000-2,499	52	17.6	82	27.8	42	14.5	26	9.0	68	23.5	2,898
	2,500-2,999	38	3.5	60	5.5	26	2.4	53	4.9	79	7.2	10,920
	3,000-3,499	53	2.3	80	3.5	42	1.9	70	3.1	112	5.0	22,534
	3,500 and over	29	1.3	47	2.2	25	1.2	50	2.3	75	3.5	21,466
	Not stated	2	30.3	17	257.6	17	265.6	1	15.6	18	281.2	64
East Anglian	**All weights**	**111**	**4.5**	**190**	**7.7**	**101**	**4.1**	**96**	**3.9**	**197**	**8.0**	**24,592**
	Under 2,500	78	50.0	127	81.4	62	41.8	23	15.5	85	57.3	1,483
	Under 1,500	43	185.3	70	301.7	36	190.5	9	47.6	45	238.1	189
	1,500-1,999	16	51.3	27	86.5	15	50.7	7	23.6	22	74.3	296
	2,000-2,499	19	18.7	30	29.5	11	11.0	7	7.0	18	18.0	998
	2,500-2,999	12	3.0	21	5.2	12	3.0	17	4.2	29	7.2	4,035
	3,000-3,499	13	1.4	25	2.7	16	1.7	31	3.3	47	5.0	9,312
	3,500 and over	7	0.7	16	1.6	11	1.1	25	2.6	36	3.7	9,736
	Not stated	1	37.0	1	37.0	-	-	-	-	-	-	26
North West Thames	**All weights**	**230**	**4.8**	**414**	**8.6**	**232**	**4.8**	**179**	**3.7**	**411**	**8.5**	**48,124**
	Under 2,500	129	36.4	250	70.5	146	42.7	48	14.0	194	56.8	3,418
	Under 1,500	50	97.8	133	260.3	98	212.6	21	45.6	119	258.1	461
	1,500-1,999	35	50.1	48	68.8	18	27.1	11	16.6	29	43.7	663
	2,000-2,499	44	18.8	69	29.5	30	13.1	16	7.0	46	20.1	2,294
	2,500-2,999	41	4.4	65	7.0	33	3.6	45	4.9	78	8.5	9,190
	3,000-3,499	32	1.7	53	2.9	28	1.5	49	2.6	77	4.2	18,501
	3,500 and over	26	1.5	40	2.4	21	1.2	35	2.1	56	3.3	16,945
	Not stated	2	27.8	6	83.3	4	57.1	2	28.6	6	85.7	70

* Including births and deaths to persons normally resident outside England and Wales.
† See Definitions, page 4.

Table 7d - *continued*

Regional health authority of residence	Birthweight (grams)	Stillbirths		Perinatal deaths		Neonatal deaths		Postneonatal deaths		Infant deaths		Live births
		Number	Rate	Number	Rate	Number	Rate	Number	Rate	Number	Rate	Number
North East Thames	**All weights**	**283**	**5.3**	**507**	**9.5**	**280**	**5.3**	**202**	**3.8**	**482**	**9.1**	**52,959**
	Under 2,500	182	45.2	334	82.9	184	47.9	66	17.2	250	65.0	3,845
	Under 1,500	98	159.3	199	323.6	121	234.0	25	48.4	146	282.4	517
	1,500-1,999	42	55.1	67	87.9	33	45.8	14	*19.4*	47	65.3	720
	2,000-2,499	42	15.8	68	25.7	30	11.5	27	10.4	57	21.9	2,608
	2,500-2,999	33	3.1	60	5.7	35	3.3	34	3.2	69	6.6	10,474
	3,000-3,499	39	1.9	62	3.0	36	1.8	55	2.7	91	4.5	20,449
	3,500 and over	28	1.5	39	2.1	14	*0.8*	47	2.6	61	3.4	18,123
	Not stated	1	*14.5*	12	*173.9*	11	*161.8*	-	-	11	*161.8*	68
South East Thames	**All weights**	**261**	**5.5**	**407**	**8.5**	**195**	**4.1**	**209**	**4.4**	**404**	**8.5**	**47,558**
	Under 2,500	152	45.1	258	76.5	137	42.5	40	12.4	177	54.9	3,222
	Under 1,500	74	143.1	145	280.5	97	219.0	14	*31.6*	111	250.6	443
	1,500-1,999	39	58.1	57	84.9	20	31.6	11	*17.4*	31	49.1	632
	2,000-2,499	39	17.8	56	25.6	20	9.3	15	*7.0*	35	16.3	2,147
	2,500-2,999	46	5.4	57	6.7	17	2.0	52	6.2	69	8.2	8,436
	3,000-3,499	34	1.9	44	2.4	15	*0.8*	64	3.5	79	4.4	18,060
	3,500 and over	28	1.6	39	2.2	16	*0.9*	53	3.0	69	3.9	17,774
	Not stated	1	*14.9*	9	*134.3*	10	*151.5*	-	-	10	*151.5*	66
South West Thames	**All weights**	**171**	**4.6**	**301**	**8.2**	**166**	**4.5**	**164**	**4.5**	**330**	**9.0**	**36,734**
	Under 2,500	105	42.1	199	79.8	109	45.6	53	22.2	162	67.8	2,388
	Under 1,500	49	126.3	114	293.8	79	233.0	26	76.7	105	309.7	339
	1,500-1,999	24	49.5	41	84.5	18	*39.0*	12	*26.0*	30	65.1	461
	2,000-2,499	32	19.8	44	27.2	12	7.6	15	*9.4*	27	17.0	1,588
	2,500-2,999	23	3.6	37	5.8	21	3.3	28	4.4	49	7.7	6,397
	3,000-3,499	25	1.8	36	2.5	21	1.5	57	4.0	78	5.5	14,111
	3,500 and over	18	*1.3*	26	1.9	12	*0.9*	25	1.8	37	2.7	13,815
	Not stated	-	-	3	*130.4*	3	*130.4*	1	*43.5*	4	*173.9*	23
Wessex	**All weights**	**187**	**5.2**	**316**	**8.8**	**171**	**4.8**	**144**	**4.0**	**315**	**8.8**	**35,772**
	Under 2,500	119	50.6	207	88.0	107	47.9	30	13.4	137	61.4	2,233
	Under 1,500	57	148.4	128	333.3	85	259.9	10	*30.6*	95	290.5	327
	1,500-1,999	31	65.5	43	90.9	14	*31.7*	11	*24.9*	25	56.6	442
	2,000-2,499	31	20.7	36	24.1	8	5.5	9	*6.1*	17	*11.6*	1,464
	2,500-2,999	34	5.7	43	7.2	17	2.9	26	4.4	43	7.3	5,903
	3,000-3,499	17	*1.2*	31	2.3	24	1.8	43	3.2	67	4.9	13,639
	3,500 and over	17	*1.2*	31	2.2	19	*1.4*	45	3.2	64	4.6	13,966
	Not stated	-	-	4	*129.0*	4	*129.0*	-	-	4	*129.0*	31
Oxford	**All weights**	**147**	**4.4**	**294**	**8.8**	**173**	**5.2**	**116**	**3.5**	**289**	**8.7**	**33,201**
	Under 2,500	96	42.1	196	85.9	109	49.9	27	12.4	136	62.2	2,186
	Under 1,500	46	150.8	114	373.8	75	289.6	5	*19.3*	80	308.9	259
	1,500-1,999	29	63.7	48	105.5	20	46.9	13	*30.5*	33	77.5	426
	2,000-2,499	21	13.8	34	22.3	14	9.3	9	*6.0*	23	15.3	1,501
	2,500-2,999	20	3.3	35	5.8	21	3.5	26	4.3	47	7.8	6,040
	3,000-3,499	16	*1.3*	31	2.4	18	*1.4*	38	3.0	56	4.4	12,676
	3,500 and over	12	*1.0*	26	2.1	22	1.8	25	2.0	47	3.8	12,221
	Not stated	3	*37.0*	6	*74.1*	3	*38.5*	-	-	3	*38.5*	78
South Western	**All weights**	**212**	**5.5**	**363**	**9.5**	**176**	**4.6**	**186**	**4.9**	**362**	**9.5**	**38,119**
	Under 2,500	133	53.7	228	92.1	112	47.8	42	17.9	154	65.8	2,342
	Under 1,500	73	206.8	140	396.6	81	289.3	14	*50.0*	95	339.3	280
	1,500-1,999	24	45.6	41	77.9	19	*37.8*	13	*25.9*	32	63.7	502
	2,000-2,499	36	22.6	47	29.4	12	7.7	15	*9.6*	27	17.3	1,560
	2,500-2,999	32	4.9	48	7.4	19	2.9	39	6.0	58	9.0	6,473
	3,000-3,499	27	1.8	48	3.3	21	1.4	68	4.6	89	6.1	14,676
	3,500 and over	16	*1.1*	27	1.8	16	*1.1*	37	2.5	53	3.6	14,589
	Not stated	4	*93.0*	12	*279.1*	8	*205.1*	-	-	8	*205.1*	39
West Midlands	**All weights**	**425**	**6.0**	**771**	**10.9**	**406**	**5.8**	**287**	**4.1**	**693**	**9.8**	**70,408**
	Under 2,500	283	50.8	537	96.4	280	53.0	73	13.8	353	66.8	5,287
	Under 1,500	147	181.0	321	395.3	187	281.2	20	30.1	207	311.3	665
	1,500-1,999	66	60.9	109	100.6	48	47.2	21	20.6	69	67.8	1,017
	2,000-2,499	70	19.0	107	29.1	45	12.5	32	8.9	77	21.4	3,605
	2,500-2,999	64	4.8	93	7.0	46	3.5	70	5.3	116	8.8	13,257
	3,000-3,499	37	1.4	67	2.5	38	1.4	85	3.2	123	4.6	26,744
	3,500 and over	40	1.6	64	2.5	33	1.3	59	2.4	92	3.7	25,078
	Not stated	1	*23.3*	10	*232.6*	9	*214.3*	-	-	9	*214.3*	42

Table 7d - *continued*

Regional health authority of residence	Birthweight (grams)	Stillbirths		Perinatal deaths		Neonatal deaths		Postneonatal deaths		Infant deaths		Live births
		Number	Rate	Number	Rate	Number	Rate	Number	Rate	Number	Rate	Number
Mersey	All weights	180	5.5	299	9.1	157	4.8	146	4.5	303	9.3	32,712
	Under 2,500	108	48.4	191	85.5	106	49.9	34	16.0	140	65.9	2,125
	Under 1,500	66	175.5	121	321.8	68	219.4	8	25.8	76	245.2	310
	1,500-1,999	20	46.3	35	81.0	21	51.0	9	21.8	30	72.8	412
	2,000-2,499	22	15.4	35	24.6	17	12.1	17	12.1	34	24.2	1,403
	2,500-2,999	31	5.7	41	7.6	18	3.4	25	4.7	43	8.0	5,366
	3,000-3,499	23	1.9	34	2.8	14	1.2	48	3.9	62	5.1	12,173
	3,500 and over	17	1.3	28	2.1	15	1.2	39	3.0	54	4.1	13,029
	Not stated	1	50.0	5	250.0	4	210.5	-	-	4	210.5	19
North Western	All weights	322	5.8	575	10.3	308	5.5	278	5.0	586	10.5	55,567
	Under 2,500	193	45.0	385	89.8	224	54.7	75	18.3	299	73.1	4,093
	Under 1,500	93	143.5	245	378.1	170	306.3	26	46.8	196	353.2	555
	1,500-1,999	40	47.7	63	75.2	32	40.1	18	22.6	50	62.7	798
	2,000-2,499	60	21.4	77	27.5	22	8.0	31	11.3	53	19.3	2,740
	2,500-2,999	53	5.0	72	6.8	24	2.3	64	6.1	88	8.4	10,509
	3,000-3,499	49	2.3	72	3.4	33	1.6	65	3.1	98	4.6	21,229
	3,500 and over	21	1.1	34	1.7	20	1.0	72	3.7	92	4.7	19,711
	Not stated	6	193.5	12	387.1	7	280.0	2	80.0	9	360.0	25

Table 8a Stillbirths - numbers and rates per 1,000 total births: age of mother x country of birth of mother; 1986   **England and Wales**

Country of birth of mother	All ages		Under 20		20-24		25-29		30-34		35 and over	
	Number	Rate	Number	Rate	Number	Rate	Number	Rate	Number	Rate	Number	Rate
All	3,549	5.3	367	6.4	1,017	5.3	1,098	4.8	680	5.2	387	7.2
United Kingdom	3,036	5.2	345	6.4	909	5.2	931	4.6	552	5.1	299	6.9
Irish Republic	28	4.5	1	4.0	6	5.9	5	2.7	7	3.7	9	7.5
Australia, Canada, New Zealand	10	4.0	1	7.9	1	2.4	6	6.7	1	1.4	1	3.1
New Commonwealth and Pakistan	373	7.0	16	6.9	80	6.1	127	6.6	93	7.2	57	10.2
New Commonwealth												
Bangladesh	31	6.5	3	5.6	7	4.9	2	1.9	8	8.5	11	13.8
India	67	6.3	1	3.2	16	4.7	30	7.5	14	6.4	6	7.0
East Africa	49	6.9	1	9.0	8	6.2	26	8.4	9	4.5	5	8.1
Rest of Africa	25	6.5	-	-	3	4.0	11	6.8	7	7.2	4	9.2
Caribbean Commonwealth	41	8.7	3	42.9	4	8.7	12	6.4	13	8.0	9	13.4
Mediterranean Commonwealth	11	3.9	1	9.4	5	7.1	2	1.7	3	5.2	-	-
Remainder of New Commonwealth	12	2.2	-	-	3	2.7	3	1.5	4	2.4	2	3.6
Pakistan	137	10.0	7	7.4	34	8.4	41	9.3	35	12.0	20	14.3
Remainder of Europe	41	4.8	2	4.9	11	5.8	10	3.8	14	6.1	4	3.2
Not stated	6	54.1	2	133.3	1	27.8	3	85.7	-	-	-	-
Other	55	4.6	-	-	9	3.6	16	4.2	13	3.9	17	9.1

Table 8b Stillbirths - numbers and rates per 1,000 total births: parity (legitimate only) x country of birth of mother; 1986   **England and Wales**

| Country of birth of mother | All | | Parity of mother (legitimate only) | | | | | | | | | | Illegitimate | |
| | | | All | | 0 | | 1 | | 2 | | 3 and over | | | |
	Number	Rate	Number	Rate	Number	Rate	Number	Rate	Number	Rate	Number	Rate	Number	Rate
All	3,549	5.3	2,600	5.0	1,141	5.5	731	3.9	403	4.9	325	7.3	949	6.7
United Kingdom	3,036	5.2	2,146	4.8	980	5.4	643	3.9	334	4.8	189	6.1	890	6.7
Irish Republic	28	4.5	22	4.6	9	6.1	4	2.6	2	2.1	7	8.4	6	4.3
Australia, Canada, New Zealand	10	4.0	8	3.8	6	5.8	1	1.4	1	3.9	-	-	2	5.1
New Commonwealth and Pakistan	373	7.0	340	7.0	115	7.8	52	3.7	52	5.9	121	10.9	33	7.4
New Commonwealth														
Bangladesh	31	6.5	31	6.5	7	8.7	3	3.7	2	2.7	19	8.0	-	-
India	67	6.3	65	6.2	26	7.5	11	3.2	17	7.9	11	7.5	2	11.2
East Africa	49	6.9	48	7.0	28	10.2	11	4.3	3	2.7	6	13.5	1	4.3
Rest of Africa	25	6.5	21	7.0	6	5.5	5	5.4	5	9.4	5	11.4	4	4.8
Caribbean Commonwealth	41	8.7	19	7.8	3	4.2	5	6.0	4	8.0	7	17.9	22	9.7
Mediterranean Commonwealth	11	3.9	10	4.0	6	6.7	2	2.2	2	4.1	-	-	1	3.2
Remainder of New Commonwealth	12	2.2	10	2.0	7	3.2	2	1.1	-	-	1	3.6	2	4.0
Pakistan	137	10.0	136	10.0	32	10.8	13	4.9	19	7.6	72	13.1	1	11.0
Remainder of Europe	41	4.8	33	4.6	15	5.1	9	3.4	7	6.7	2	4.3	8	5.9
Not stated	6	54.1	-	-	-	-	-	-	-	-	-	-	6	240.0
Other	55	4.6	51	4.6	16	3.6	22	5.9	7	4.2	6	5.5	4	4.7

Table 9a Perinatal deaths - numbers and rates per 1,000 total births: age of mother x country of birth of mother; 1986   England and Wales

Country of birth of mother	All ages Number	Rate	Under 20 Number	Rate	20-24 Number	Rate	25-29 Number	Rate	30-34 Number	Rate	35 and over Number	Rate
All	6,338	9.5	728	12.6	1,823	9.4	1,948	8.5	1,172	9.0	667	12.5
United Kingdom	5,469	9.4	679	12.5	1,633	9.4	1,665	8.3	960	8.8	532	12.3
Irish Republic	51	8.2	3	11.9	10	9.9	12	6.4	12	6.4	14	11.7
Australia, Canada, New Zealand	19	7.7	2	15.9	3	7.2	10	11.1	3	4.2	1	3.1
New Commonwealth and Pakistan	624	11.8	34	14.8	142	10.8	209	10.9	152	11.8	87	15.6
New Commonwealth												
Bangladesh	46	9.7	5	9.4	10	7.0	4	3.8	11	11.6	16	20.1
India	113	10.5	2	6.5	25	7.4	45	11.3	27	12.4	14	16.3
East Africa	84	11.9	3	27.0	16	12.5	39	12.6	19	9.6	7	11.4
Rest of Africa	40	10.4	-	-	7	9.3	18	11.2	8	8.2	7	16.1
Caribbean Commonwealth	59	12.5	5	71.4	5	10.8	18	9.5	20	12.3	11	16.4
Mediterranean Commonwealth	25	8.9	1	9.4	11	15.6	6	5.2	5	8.7	2	7.8
Remainder of New Commonwealth	26	4.7	-	-	8	7.2	8	4.0	8	4.8	2	3.6
Pakistan	231	16.9	18	19.0	60	14.8	71	16.1	54	18.6	28	20.1
Remainder of Europe	67	7.9	5	12.2	17	9.0	17	6.5	19	8.3	9	7.2
Not stated	9	81.1	3	200.0	2	55.6	4	114.3	-	-	-	-
Other	99	8.4	2	5.6	16	6.4	31	8.2	26	7.8	24	12.8

Table 9b Perinatal deaths - numbers and rates per 1,000 total births: parity (legitimate only) x country of birth of mother; 1986   England and Wales

Country of birth of mother	All Number	Rate	Parity (All) Number	Rate	0 Number	Rate	1 Number	Rate	2 Number	Rate	3 and over Number	Rate	Illegitimate Number	Rate
All	6,338	9.5	4,591	8.8	1,971	9.5	1,379	7.3	697	8.5	544	12.2	1,747	12.3
United Kingdom	5,469	9.4	3,826	8.5	1,720	9.5	1,193	7.2	568	8.2	345	11.2	1,643	12.3
Irish Republic	51	8.2	36	7.5	12	8.2	8	5.1	8	8.4	8	9.7	15	10.8
Australia, Canada, New Zealand	19	7.7	15	7.2	9	8.7	4	5.7	2	7.7	-	-	4	10.2
New Commonwealth and Pakistan	624	11.8	567	11.7	180	12.1	115	8.2	96	11.0	176	15.9	57	12.8
New Commonwealth														
Bangladesh	46	9.7	46	9.7	8	9.9	8	10.0	5	6.8	25	10.5	-	-
India	113	10.5	111	10.5	33	9.6	30	8.7	29	13.5	19	12.9	2	11.2
East Africa	84	11.9	81	11.8	41	15.0	19	7.4	5	4.6	16	35.9	3	12.9
Rest of Africa	40	10.4	30	10.0	10	9.1	7	7.5	6	11.3	7	16.0	10	12.0
Caribbean Commonwealth	59	12.5	26	10.7	4	5.6	9	10.8	4	8.0	9	23.1	33	14.5
Mediterranean Commonwealth	25	8.9	20	8.0	11	12.3	5	5.4	3	6.1	1	5.5	5	15.8
Remainder of New Commonwealth	26	4.7	23	4.6	12	5.5	7	3.9	2	2.8	2	7.2	3	6.0
Pakistan	231	16.9	230	16.9	61	20.6	30	11.4	42	16.7	97	17.7	1	11.0
Remainder of Europe	67	7.9	55	7.7	24	8.1	22	8.3	7	6.7	2	4.3	12	8.9
Not stated	9	81.1	-	-	-	-	-	-	-	-	-	-	9	360.0
Other	99	8.4	92	8.4	26	5.8	37	9.9	16	9.6	13	11.9	7	8.2

Table 10a Neonatal deaths - numbers and rates per 1,000 live births: England and Wales
age of mother x country of birth of mother; 1986

Country of birth of mother	Age of mother											
	All ages		Under 20		20-24		25-29		30-34		35 and over	
	Number	Rate	Number	Rate	Number	Rate	Number	Rate	Number	Rate	Number	Rate
All	3,449	5.2	435	7.6	1,009	5.3	1,074	4.7	597	4.6	334	6.3
United Kingdom	2,992	5.2	403	7.5	902	5.2	924	4.6	493	4.5	270	6.3
Irish Republic	26	4.2	2	7.9	4	4.0	9	4.8	6	3.2	5	4.2
Australia, Canada, New Zealand	10	4.0	1	8.0	3	7.3	4	4.5	2	2.8	-	-
New Commonwealth and Pakistan	330	6.3	23	10.1	81	6.2	108	5.7	76	6.0	42	7.6
New Commonwealth												
Bangladesh	23	4.9	3	5.7	3	2.1	4	3.8	4	4.3	9	11.5
India	54	5.1	1	3.2	14	4.2	15	3.8	14	6.5	10	11.7
East Africa	51	7.2	3	27.3	11	8.6	19	6.2	15	7.6	3	4.9
Rest of Africa	20	5.3	-	-	5	6.7	10	6.2	2	2.1	3	7.0
Caribbean Commonwealth	28	6.0	2	29.9	1	2.2	10	5.3	13	8.1	2	3.0
Mediterranean Commonwealth	18	6.4	-	-	6	8.5	6	5.2	2	3.5	4	15.6
Remainder of New Commonwealth	19	3.5	2	12.0	6	5.4	6	3.0	4	2.4	1	1.8
Pakistan	117	8.6	12	12.8	35	8.7	38	8.7	22	7.6	10	7.3
Remainder of Europe	36	4.3	3	7.4	10	5.3	10	3.8	6	2.6	7	5.6
Not stated	4	38.1	1	76.9	1	28.6	2	62.5	-	-	-	-
Other	51	4.3	2	5.6	8	3.2	17	4.5	14	4.2	10	5.4

Table 10b Neonatal deaths - numbers and rates per 1,000 live births: England and Wales
parity (legitimate only) x country of birth of mother; 1986

Country of birth of mother	All		Parity of mother (legitimate only)										Illegitimate	
			All		0		1		2		3 and over			
	Number	Rate	Number	Rate	Number	Rate	Number	Rate	Number	Rate	Number	Rate	Number	Rate
All	3,449	5.2	2,461	4.7	1,025	5.0	807	4.3	365	4.5	264	6.0	988	7.0
United Kingdom	2,992	5.2	2,061	4.6	898	5.0	685	4.1	293	4.3	185	6.0	931	7.0
Irish Republic	26	4.2	17	3.5	3	2.1	4	2.6	7	7.3	3	3.6	9	6.5
Australia, Canada, New Zealand	10	4.0	8	3.8	4	3.9	3	4.2	1	3.9	-	-	2	5.1
New Commonwealth and Pakistan	330	6.3	299	6.2	96	6.5	81	5.8	54	6.2	68	6.2	31	7.0
New Commonwealth														
Bangladesh	23	4.9	23	4.9	2	2.5	6	7.5	4	5.4	11	4.6	-	-
India	54	5.1	54	5.2	11	3.2	21	6.1	14	6.6	8	5.5	-	-
East Africa	51	7.2	48	7.1	22	8.1	10	3.9	5	4.6	11	25.0	3	12.9
Rest of Africa	20	5.3	14	4.7	9	8.3	2	2.2	1	1.9	2	4.6	6	7.2
Caribbean Commonwealth	28	6.0	13	5.4	3	4.2	8	9.7	-	-	2	5.2	15	6.6
Mediterranean Commonwealth	18	6.4	14	5.6	6	6.7	5	5.4	2	4.1	1	5.5	4	12.7
Remainder of New Commonwealth	19	3.5	16	3.2	8	3.7	5	2.8	2	2.8	1	3.6	3	6.0
Pakistan	117	8.6	117	8.7	35	11.9	24	9.1	26	10.4	32	5.5	-	-
Remainder of Europe	36	4.3	28	3.9	11	3.7	16	6.0	-	-	1	2.2	8	6.0
Not stated	4	38.1	1	11.6	-	-	1	40.0	-	-	-	-	3	157.9
Other	51	4.3	47	4.3	13	2.9	17	4.6	10	6.0	7	6.5	4	4.7

Table 11a   Postneonatal deaths - numbers and rates per 1,000 live births: **England and Wales**
age of mother x country of birth of mother; 1986

Country of birth of mother	Age of mother											
	All ages		Under 20		20-24		25-29		30-34		35 and over	
	Number	Rate	Number	Rate	Number	Rate	Number	Rate	Number	Rate	Number	Rate
All	2,760	4.2	412	7.2	959	5.0	814	3.6	387	3.0	188	3.5
United Kingdom	2,438	4.2	392	7.3	864	5.0	708	3.5	321	3.0	153	3.6
Irish Republic	25	4.0	4	15.9	6	6.0	5	2.7	5	2.7	5	4.2
Australia, Canada, New Zealand	11	4.5	2	16.0	1	2.4	4	4.5	3	4.2	1	3.2
New Commonwealth and Pakistan	221	4.2	9	3.9	68	5.2	78	4.1	45	3.5	21	3.8
New Commonwealth												
Bangladesh	11	2.3	2	3.8	2	1.4	2	1.9	4	4.3	1	1.3
India	42	3.9	3	9.7	18	5.4	17	4.3	2	0.9	2	2.3
East Africa	21	3.0	-	-	5	3.9	9	2.9	6	3.0	1	1.6
Rest of Africa	18	4.7	-	-	7	9.3	8	5.0	3	3.1	-	-
Caribbean Commonwealth	20	4.3	-	-	2	4.4	10	5.3	3	1.9	5	7.6
Mediterranean Commonwealth	9	3.2	-	-	3	4.3	2	1.7	4	7.0	-	-
Remainder of New Commonwealth	17	3.1	1	6.0	3	2.7	8	4.0	4	2.4	1	1.8
Pakistan	83	6.1	3	3.2	28	7.0	22	5.0	19	6.6	11	8.0
Remainder of Europe	36	4.3	3	7.4	16	8.5	10	3.8	5	2.2	2	1.6
Not stated	1	9.5	-	-	-	-	-	-	-	-	1	111.1
Other	28	2.4	2	5.6	4	1.6	9	2.4	8	2.4	5	2.7

Table 11b   Postneonatal deaths - numbers and rates per 1,000 live births: **England and Wales**
parity (legitimate only) x country of birth of mother; 1986

Country of birth of mother	All		Parity of mother (legitimate only)										Illegitimate	
			All		0		1		2		3 and over			
	Number	Rate	Number	Rate	Number	Rate	Number	Rate	Number	Rate	Number	Rate	Number	Rate
All	2,760	4.2	1,901	3.7	538	2.6	725	3.8	405	5.0	233	5.3	859	6.1
United Kingdom	2,438	4.2	1,631	3.7	460	2.5	642	3.9	358	5.2	171	5.6	807	6.1
Irish Republic	25	4.0	14	2.9	3	2.1	5	3.2	5	5.2	1	1.2	11	7.9
Australia,Canada, New Zealand	11	4.5	7	3.4	5	4.9	1	1.4	1	3.9	-	-	4	10.3
New Commonwealth and Pakistan	221	4.2	199	4.1	52	3.5	58	4.2	33	3.8	56	5.1	22	5.0
New Commonwealth														
Bangladesh	11	2.3	11	2.3	2	2.5	3	3.8	1	1.4	5	2.1	-	-
India	42	3.9	42	4.0	15	4.4	12	3.5	8	3.7	7	4.8	-	-
East Africa	21	3.0	20	2.9	7	2.6	8	3.1	4	3.7	1	2.3	1	4.3
Rest of Africa	18	4.7	12	4.0	5	4.6	5	5.4	2	3.8	-	-	6	7.2
Caribbean Commonwealth	20	4.3	9	3.7	2	2.8	4	4.8	-	-	3	7.8	11	4.9
Mediterranean Commonwealth	9	3.2	9	3.6	3	3.4	5	5.4	-	-	1	5.5	-	-
Remainder of New Commonwealth	17	3.1	13	2.6	5	2.3	3	1.7	3	4.1	2	7.2	4	8.0
Pakistan	83	6.1	83	6.2	13	4.4	18	6.9	15	6.0	37	6.8	-	-
Remainder of Europe	36	4.3	23	3.2	10	3.4	10	3.8	2	1.9	1	2.2	13	9.7
Not stated	1	9.5	1	11.6	-	-	1	40.0	-	-	-	-	-	-
Other	28	2.4	26	2.4	8	1.8	8	2.2	6	3.6	4	3.7	2	2.3

Table 12a Infant deaths - numbers and rates per 1,000 live births: age of mother x country of birth of mother; 1986 **England and Wales**

Country of birth of mother	All ages		Under 20		20-24		25-29		30-34		35 and over	
	Number	Rate	Number	Rate	Number	Rate	Number	Rate	Number	Rate	Number	Rate
All	6,209	9.4	847	14.8	1,968	10.2	1,888	8.2	984	7.6	522	9.8
United Kingdom	5,430	9.4	795	14.7	1,766	10.2	1,632	8.1	814	7.5	423	9.9
Irish Republic	51	8.2	6	23.8	10	9.9	14	7.5	11	5.9	10	8.4
Australia, Canada, New Zealand	21	8.5	3	24.0	4	9.7	8	8.9	5	7.0	1	3.2
New Commonwealth and Pakistan	551	10.5	32	14.0	149	11.4	186	9.8	121	9.5	63	11.4
New Commonwealth												
Bangladesh	34	7.2	5	9.5	5	3.5	6	5.7	8	8.5	10	12.7
India	96	9.0	4	12.9	32	9.5	32	8.1	16	7.4	12	14.1
East Africa	72	10.2	3	27.3	16	12.6	28	9.1	21	10.7	4	6.6
Rest of Africa	38	10.0	-	-	12	16.0	18	11.2	5	5.2	3	7.0
Caribbean Commonwealth	48	10.3	2	29.9	3	6.6	20	10.7	16	9.9	7	10.6
Mediterranean Commonwealth	27	9.7	-	-	9	12.8	8	6.9	6	10.5	4	15.6
Remainder of New Commonwealth	36	6.6	3	18.0	9	8.2	14	7.0	8	4.9	2	3.6
Pakistan	200	14.8	15	15.9	63	15.7	60	13.8	41	14.3	21	15.3
Remainder of Europe	72	8.5	6	14.7	26	13.8	20	7.6	11	4.8	9	7.2
Not stated	5	47.6	1	76.9	1	28.6	2	62.5	-	-	1	111.1
Other	79	6.7	4	11.2	12	4.8	26	6.9	22	6.6	15	8.1

Table 12b Infant deaths - numbers and rates per 1,000 live births: parity (legitimate only) x country of birth of mother; 1986 **England and Wales**

Country of birth of mother	All		Parity of mother (legitimate only)												Illegitimate	
			All		0		1		2		3 and over					
	Number	Rate	Number	Rate	Number	Rate	Number	Rate	Number	Rate	Number	Rate			Number	Rate
All	6,209	9.4	4,362	8.4	1,563	7.6	1,532	8.1	770	9.5	497	11.3			1,847	13.1
United Kingdom	5,430	9.4	3,692	8.3	1,358	7.5	1,327	8.0	651	9.5	356	11.6			1,738	13.1
Irish Republic	51	8.2	31	6.5	6	4.1	9	5.8	12	12.6	4	4.9			20	14.4
Australia, Canada, New Zealand	21	8.5	15	7.2	9	8.8	4	5.7	2	7.8	-	-			6	15.4
New Commonwealth and Pakistan	551	10.5	498	10.3	148	10.1	139	10.0	87	10.0	124	11.3			53	12.0
New Commonwealth																
Bangladesh	34	7.2	34	7.2	4	5.0	9	11.3	5	6.8	16	6.8			-	-
India	96	9.0	96	9.2	26	7.6	33	9.6	22	10.3	15	10.2			-	-
East Africa	72	10.2	68	10.0	29	10.7	18	7.0	9	8.2	12	27.3			4	17.2
Rest of Africa	38	10.0	26	8.7	14	12.9	7	7.5	3	5.7	2	4.6			12	14.4
Caribbean Commonwealth	48	10.3	22	9.1	5	7.1	12	14.5	-	-	5	13.1			26	11.5
Mediterranean Commonwealth	27	9.7	23	9.3	9	10.1	10	10.9	2	4.1	2	11.0			4	12.7
Remainder of New Commonwealth	36	6.6	29	5.8	13	6.0	8	4.4	5	6.9	3	10.8			7	14.0
Pakistan	200	14.8	200	14.8	48	16.4	42	16.0	41	16.5	69	12.7			-	-
Remainder of Europe	72	8.5	51	7.2	21	7.2	26	9.8	2	1.9	2	4.3			21	15.7
Not stated	5	47.6	2	23.3	-	-	2	80.0	-	-	-	-			3	157.9
Other	79	6.7	73	6.7	21	4.7	25	6.7	16	9.6	11	10.1			6	7.0

Table 13a   Live births - numbers: England and Wales
             age of mother x country of birth of mother; 1986

Country of birth of mother	Age of mother					
	All ages	Under 20	20-24	25-29	30-34	35 and over
All	661,018	57,406	192,064	229,035	129,487	53,026
United Kingdom	579,322	53,963	173,173	200,795	108,524	42,867
Irish Republic	6,188	252	1,008	1,868	1,869	1,191
Australia, Canada, New Zealand	2,470	125	413	896	719	317
New Commonwealth and Pakistan	52,705	2,287	13,073	19,062	12,751	5,532
New Commonwealth						
Bangladesh	4,717	529	1,416	1,048	938	786
India	10,650	309	3,362	3,959	2,167	853
East Africa	7,037	110	1,274	3,073	1,971	609
Rest of Africa	3,805	59	749	1,601	966	430
Caribbean Commonwealth	4,674	67	458	1,875	1,612	662
Mediterranean Commonwealth	2,795	105	702	1,157	574	257
Remainder of New Commonwealth	5,468	167	1,104	1,990	1,647	560
Pakistan	13,559	941	4,008	4,359	2,876	1,375
Remainder of Europe	8,435	408	1,880	2,622	2,274	1,251
Not stated	105	13	35	32	16	9
Other	11,793	358	2,482	3,760	3,334	1,859

Table 13b   Live births - numbers: England and Wales
             parity (legitimate) x country of birth of mother

Country of birth of mother	All	Parity of mother (legitimate only)					Illegitimate
		All	0	1	2	3 and over	
All	661,018	519,673	205,586	188,539	81,460	44,088	141,345
United Kingdom	579,322	446,383	180,929	165,963	68,835	30,656	132,939
Irish Republic	6,188	4,799	1,460	1,563	954	822	1,389
Australia, Canada, New Zealand	2,470	2,081	1,024	706	258	93	389
New Commonwealth and Pakistan	52,705	48,289	14,708	13,917	8,697	10,967	4,416
New Commonwealth							
Bangladesh	4,717	4,702	798	800	738	2,366	15
India	10,650	10,474	3,428	3,446	2,136	1,464	176
East Africa	7,037	6,805	2,712	2,558	1,095	440	232
Rest of Africa	3,805	2,973	1,087	928	525	433	832
Caribbean Commonwealth	4,674	2,418	708	828	499	383	2,256
Mediterranean Commonwealth	2,795	2,479	889	920	489	181	316
Remainder of New Commonwealth	5,468	4,969	2,156	1,813	723	277	499
Pakistan	13,559	13,469	2,930	2,624	2,492	5,423	90
Remainder of Europe	8,435	7,095	2,935	2,657	1,039	464	1,340
Not stated	105	86	43	25	16	2	19
Other	11,793	10,940	4,487	3,708	1,661	1,084	853

Table 14a   Stillbirths (a) and neonatal deaths (b) - numbers: **England and Wales**
age of mother by main cause of death, 1986

ICD number	Cause of death			Age of mother							
				All ages	Under 20	20-24	25-29	30-34	35-39	40-44	45 and over
	All causes	Stillbirths	(a)	3,549	367	1,017	1,098	680	315	63	9
		Neonatal deaths	(b)	3,449	435	1,009	1,074	597	288	44	2
	Fetal mentions		(a)	2,715	283	758	847	540	231	44	12
			(b)	4,368	549	1,271	1,381	749	359	56	3
740-759	Congenital anomalies		(a)	283	26	75	85	63	21	9	4
			(b)	1,230	133	342	415	211	110	18	1
740	Anencephalus		(a)	41	5	13	7	10	5	1	-
			(b)	26	5	6	11	3	-	1	-
741	Spina bifida		(a)	21	3	7	8	2	1	-	-
			(b)	65	6	22	24	10	3	-	-
7420	Encephalocele		(a)	1	-	-	-	-	1	-	-
			(b)	26	5	7	10	2	2	-	-
742 rem	Other congenital anomalies of central nervous system		(a)	42	4	12	12	9	1	3	1
			(b)	65	8	20	21	11	4	1	-
745	Bulbus cordis anomalies and anomalies of cardiac septal closure		(a)	2	-	1	-	-	-	1	-
			(b)	115	6	25	47	24	10	3	-
746	Other congenital anomalies of heart		(a)	10	-	4	3	2	1	-	-
			(b)	224	23	72	66	42	18	3	-
747	Other congenital anomalies of circulatory system		(a)	1	-	-	1	-	-	-	-
			(b)	103	13	26	37	15	12	-	-
748	Congenital anomalies of respiratory system		(a)	7	1	1	1	3	1	-	-
			(b)	163	23	41	57	27	15	-	-
749-751	Cleft palate and lip; other congenital anomalies of upper alimentary tract and digestive system		(a)	12	-	1	5	3	2	-	1
			(b)	43	3	6	22	8	4	-	-
753	Congenital anomalies of urinary system		(a)	31	2	5	12	11	1	-	-
			(b)	101	10	31	37	15	8	-	-
754-756	Congenital musculoskeletal anomalies		(a)	33	1	7	16	7	1	-	1
			(b)	124	9	37	34	25	15	4	-
758	Chromosomal anomalies		(a)	21	1	5	5	5	3	2	-
			(b)	73	7	20	17	14	10	4	1
740-759 rem	Other and unspecified congenital anomalies		(a)	61	9	19	15	11	4	2	1
			(b)	102	15	29	32	15	9	2	-
764,765	Prematurity		(a)	181	24	50	52	30	19	5	1
			(b)	882	144	244	249	147	82	15	1
764	Slow fetal growth and fetal malnutrition		(a)	147	17	47	42	21	15	4	1
			(b)	12	1	3	5	2	1	-	-
765	Disorders relating to short gestation and unspecified low birthweight		(a)	34	7	3	10	9	4	1	-
			(b)	870	143	241	244	145	81	15	1
7650	Extreme immaturity		(a)	3	1	-	-	-	1	1	-
			(b)	634	109	172	178	102	63	10	-
7651	Other preterm infants		(a)	31	6	3	10	9	3	-	-
			(b)	236	34	69	66	43	18	5	1
767	Birth trauma		(a)	12	-	7	4	-	1	-	-
			(b)	87	13	27	32	9	5	1	-
7670	Subdural and cerebral haemorrhage		(a)	12	-	7	4	-	1	-	-
			(b)	77	10	22	30	9	5	1	-

Table 14a - *continued*

ICD number	Cause of death		All ages	Under 20	20-24	25-29	30-34	35-39	40-44	45 and over
										Age of mother
768	Intrauterine hypoxia and birth asphyxia	(a)	1,135	112	320	372	229	88	11	3
		(b)	325	25	98	113	67	19	2	1
7680	Death from asphyxia or anoxia before onset of labour or at unspecified time	(a)	930	93	260	301	186	77	10	3
		(b)	-	-	-	-	-	-	-	-
7681	Death from asphyxia or anoxia during labour	(a)	205	19	60	71	43	11	1	-
		(b)	-	-	-	-	-	-	-	-
7689	Unspecified birth asphyxia in liveborn infant	(a)	-	-	-	-	-	-	-	-
		(b)	180	12	60	60	36	10	2	-
512,514, 516,518, 519,769, 770	Non-infectious respiratory disorders	(a)	10	1	4	3	1	1	-	-
		(b)	904	123	292	272	143	68	6	-
769	Respiratory distress syndrome	(a)	-	-	-	-	-	-	-	-
		(b)	475	59	168	139	69	36	4	-
770	Other respiratory conditions of fetus and newborn	(a)	10	1	4	3	1	1	-	-
		(b)	426	64	123	131	74	32	2	-
001-139, 320-326, 460-511, 513,771	Infections and infectious diseases	(a)	10	2	3	2	2	1	-	-
		(b)	199	24	47	58	53	14	3	-
320-322	Meningitis	(a)	-	-	-	-	-	-	-	-
		(b)	26	4	3	7	8	3	1	-
480-486	Pneumonia	(a)	-	-	-	-	-	-	-	-
		(b)	47	5	15	11	14	2	-	-
771	Infections specific to the perinatal period	(a)	10	2	3	2	2	1	-	-
		(b)	108	11	27	34	26	8	2	-
766, 772-779	Other perinatal causes	(a)	441	42	122	142	90	37	7	1
		(b)	455	55	127	157	74	37	5	-
766	Disorders relating to long gestation and high birthweight	(a)	9	3	1	4	1	-	-	-
		(b)	3	1	-	1	1	-	-	-
772	Fetal and neonatal haemorrhage	(a)	14	2	5	2	3	2	-	-
		(b)	226	32	64	78	37	12	3	-
773	Haemolytic disease of fetus or newborn, due to isoimmunization	(a)	16	-	4	3	5	2	2	-
		(b)	14	-	4	5	-	5	-	-
7730	due to Rh isoimmunization	(a)	10	-	2	2	3	1	2	-
		(b)	6	-	2	1	-	3	-	-
774	Other perinatal jaundice	(a)	-	-	-	-	-	-	-	-
		(b)	1	1	-	-	-	-	-	-
775	Endocrine and metabolic disturbances specific to the fetus and newborn	(a)	6	1	3	1	1	-	-	-
		(b)	5	-	2	2	-	1	-	-
7750	Syndrome of 'infant of a diabetic mother'	(a)	6	1	3	1	1	-	-	-
		(b)	-	-	-	-	-	-	-	-
776	Haematological disorders of fetus and newborn	(a)	2	-	1	1	-	-	-	-
		(b)	16	1	2	8	3	1	1	-
777	Perinatal disorders of digestive system	(a)	-	-	-	-	-	-	-	-
		(b)	54	5	11	18	14	6	-	-
778	Conditions involving the integument and temperature regulation of fetus and newborn	(a)	20	2	5	10	2	-	1	-
		(b)	30	5	8	12	2	3	-	-

Table 14a - *continued*

ICD number	Cause of death		All ages	Under 20	20-24	25-29	30-34	35-39	40-44	45 and over
										Age of mother
779	Other and ill-defined conditions originating in the perinatal period	(a) (b)	374 106	34 10	103 36	121 33	78 17	33 9	4 1	1 -
7799	Unspecified perinatal conditions	(a) (b)	363 ·	34 -	102 -	115 -	76 -	31 -	4 -	1 -
4275, 428, 584-586, 780-799, 800-999	Ill-defined conditions, modes of death, injury and poisoning	(a) (b)	2 153	- 20	- 60	1 30	1 25	- 14	- 4	- -
798	Sudden death, cause unknown	(a) (b)	· 78	- 6	- 40	- 14	- 12	- 4	- 2	- -
7980	Sudden infant death syndrome	(a) (b)	· 78	- 6	- 40	- 14	- 12	- 4	- 2	- -
760-763	Maternal conditions certified as fetal	(a) (b)	627 35	75 6	175 10	181 10	119 6	62 2	12 1	3 -
001-E999 rem	Other fetal causes	(a) (b)	14 98	1 6	2 24	5 45	5 14	1 8	- 1	- -
7996	No fetal cause	(a) (b)	1,111 5	109 1	331 1	338 1	208 2	101 -	22 -	2 -
	Maternal mentions	(a) (b)	1,342 906	133 94	390 249	408 290	256 168	124 97	27 7	4 1
642, 7600	Hypertension	(a) (b)	254 117	25 8	78 28	76 39	47 24	17 15	9 2	2 1
647,648, 760 rem	Other maternal conditions which may be unrelated to the present pregnancy	(a) (b)	30 18	4 -	7 6	5 6	10 4	3 2	1 -	- -
761	Maternal complications in pregnancy	(a) (b)	· 1	- -	- -	- 1	- -	- -	- -	- -
762	Complications of placenta, cord and membranes	(a) (b)	· ·	- -	- -	- -	- -	- -	- -	- -
651, 7615	Multiple pregnancy	(a) (b)	44 61	1 7	10 17	16 14	9 16	7 7	1 -	- -
630-639, 643,646, 650,663, 655-658, 670-676, 761-762 rem	Other maternal complications of pregnancy, placenta, cord or membranes	(a) (b)	333 232	35 20	88 55	97 83	67 47	36 24	10 3	- -
7622	Other and unspecified morphological and functional abnormalities of placenta	(a) (b)	· ·	- -	- -	- -	- -	- -	- -	- -
7624	Prolapsed cord	(a) (b)	· ·	- -	- -	- -	- -	- -	- -	- -
7625	Other compression of umbilical cord	(a) (b)	· ·	- -	- -	- -	- -	- -	- -	- -
640,641, 7620, 7621	Maternal antepartum haemorrhage	(a) (b)	506 180	55 22	165 60	167 52	78 32	37 14	3 -	1 -
7620	Placenta praevia	(a) (b)	· ·	- -	- -	- -	- -	- -	- -	- -

Table 14a - *continued*

ICD number	Cause of death		All ages	Under 20	20-24	25-29	30-34	35-39	40-44	45 and over
7621	Other forms of placental separation and haemorrhage	(a)	·	-	-	-	-	-	-	-
		(b)	·	-	-	-	-	-	-	-
644,645, 652-654, 659-662, 664-669, 7610, 7617,763	Complications of presentation, labour and delivery	(a)	45	4	10	8	10	13	-	-
		(b)	212	29	57	71	32	22	1	-
763	Other complications of labour and delivery	(a)	·	-	-	-	-	-	-	-
		(b)	1	-	-	-	-	1	-	-
001- E999 rem	Other maternal conditions	(a)	130	9	32	39	35	11	3	1
		(b)	86	8	26	25	13	13	1	-
7996	No maternal cause	(a)	2,308	251	649	721	444	200	38	5
		(b)	2,637	354	780	825	439	200	38	1
Total live births		M	338,852	29,311	98,666	117,402	66,164	23,444	3,599	266
		F	322,166	28,095	93,398	111,633	63,323	22,021	3,434	262
		P	661,018	57,406	192,064	229,035	129,487	45,465	7,033	528

31

Table 14b Stillbirths (a) and neonatal deaths (b) - rates per 1,000 total/live births: age of mother by selected cause of death, 1986   **England and Wales**

N-list number	Cause of death			All ages	Under 20	20-24	25-29	30-34	35-39	40-44	45 and over
	All causes	Stillbirth rates	(a)	5.3	6.4	5.3	4.8	5.2	6.9	8.9	16.8
		Neonatal death rates	(b)	5.2	7.6	5.3	4.7	4.6	6.3	6.3	3.8
	Fetal mentions		(a)	4.1	4.9	3.9	3.7	4.1	5.0	6.2	22.4
			(b)	6.6	9.6	6.6	6.0	5.8	7.9	8.0	5.7
N01	Anencephalus		(a)	0.1	0.1	0.1	0.0	0.1	0.1	0.1	-
			(b)	0.0	0.1	0.0	0.0	0.0	-	0.1	-
N02	Spina bifida		(a)	0.0	0.1	0.0	0.0	0.0	0.0	-	-
			(b)	0.1	0.1	0.1	0.1	0.1	0.1	-	-
N03	Encephalocele		(a)	0.0	-	-	-	-	0.0	-	-
			(b)	0.0	0.1	0.0	0.0	0.0	0.0	-	-
N04	Other congenital anomalies of central nervous system		(a)	0.1	0.1	0.1	0.1	0.1	0.0	0.4	1.9
			(b)	0.1	0.1	0.1	0.1	0.1	0.1	0.1	-
N05	Congenital anomalies of circulatory system		(a)	0.0	-	0.0	0.0	0.0	0.0	0.1	-
			(b)	0.7	0.7	0.6	0.7	0.6	0.9	0.9	-
N06	Other congenital anomalies		(a)	0.2	0.2	0.2	0.2	0.3	0.3	0.6	5.6
			(b)	0.9	1.2	0.9	0.9	0.8	1.3	1.4	1.9
N07	Prematurity		(a)	0.3	0.4	0.3	0.2	0.2	0.4	0.7	1.9
			(b)	1.3	2.5	1.3	1.1	1.1	1.8	2.1	1.9
N08	Birth trauma		(a)	0.0	-	0.0	0.0	-	0.0	-	-
			(b)	0.1	0.2	0.1	0.1	0.1	0.1	0.1	-
N09	Birth asphyxia		(a)	1.7	1.9	1.7	1.6	1.8	1.9	1.6	5.6
			(b)	0.5	0.4	0.5	0.5	0.5	0.4	0.3	1.9
N10	Non-infectious respiratory disorders		(a)	0.0	0.0	0.0	0.0	0.0	0.0	-	-
			(b)	1.4	2.1	1.5	1.2	1.1	1.5	0.9	-
N11	Infections and infectious diseases		(a)	0.0	0.0	0.0	0.0	0.0	0.0	-	-
			(b)	0.3	0.4	0.2	0.3	0.4	0.3	0.4	-
N12	Other perinatal causes		(a)	0.7	0.7	0.6	0.6	0.7	0.8	1.0	1.9
			(b)	0.7	1.0	0.7	0.7	0.6	0.8	0.7	-
N13	Ill-defined conditions, modes of death, injury and poisoning		(a)	0.0	-	-	0.0	0.0	-	-	-
			(b)	0.2	0.3	0.3	0.1	0.2	0.3	0.6	-
N14	Maternal conditions classified as fetal		(a)	0.9	1.3	0.9	0.8	0.9	1.4	1.7	5.6
			(b)	0.1	0.1	0.1	0.0	0.0	0.0	0.1	-
N15	Other fetal causes		(a)	0.0	0.0	0.0	0.0	0.0	0.0	-	-
			(b)	0.1	0.1	0.1	0.2	0.1	0.2	0.1	-
N16	No fetal cause		(a)	1.7	1.9	1.7	1.5	1.6	2.2	3.1	3.7
			(b)	0.0	0.0	0.0	0.0	0.0	-	-	-
	Maternal mentions		(a)	2.0	2.3	2.0	1.8	2.0	2.7	3.8	7.4
			(b)	1.4	1.6	1.3	1.3	1.3	2.1	1.0	1.9
N17	Hypertension		(a)	0.4	0.4	0.4	0.3	0.4	0.4	1.3	3.7
			(b)	0.2	0.1	0.1	0.2	0.2	0.3	0.3	1.9
N18	Other maternal conditions which may be unrelated to the present pregnancy		(a)	0.0	0.1	0.0	0.0	0.1	0.1	0.1	-
			(b)	0.0	-	0.0	0.0	0.0	0.0	-	-
N19	Multiple pregnancy		(a)	0.1	0.0	0.1	0.1	0.1	0.2	0.1	-
			(b)	0.1	0.1	0.1	0.1	0.1	0.2	-	-
N20	Other maternal complications related to pregnancy, placenta, cord or membranes		(a)	0.5	0.6	0.5	0.4	0.5	0.8	1.4	-
			(b)	0.4	0.3	0.3	0.4	0.4	0.5	0.4	-

Table 14b - *continued*

N-list number	Cause of death		Age of mother							
			All ages	Under 20	20-24	25-29	30-34	35-39	40-44	45 and over
N21	Maternal antepartum haemorrhage	(a)	0.8	1.0	0.9	0.7	0.6	0.8	*0.4*	*1.9*
		(b)	0.3	0.4	0.3	0.2	0.2	*0.3*	-	-
N22	Complications of presentation, labour and delivery	(a)	0.1	*0.1*	*0.1*	*0.0*	*0.1*	*0.3*	-	-
		(b)	0.3	0.5	0.3	0.3	0.2	0.5	*0.1*	-
N23	Other maternal conditions	(a)	0.2	*0.2*	0.2	0.2	0.3	*0.2*	*0.4*	*1.9*
		(b)	0.1	*0.1*	0.1	0.1	*0.1*	*0.3*	*0.1*	-
N24	No maternal cause	(a)	3.5	4.3	3.4	3.1	3.4	4.4	5.4	*9.3*
		(b)	4.0	6.2	4.1	3.6	3.4	4.4	5.4	*1.9*

Table 15 Postneonatal deaths - numbers and rates per 1,000 live births: **England and Wales**
age of mother by selected cause of death, 1986

ICD number	Cause of death	Age of mother					
		All ages	Under 20	20 - 24	25 - 29	30 - 34	35 and over
	Numbers						
	All causes	**2,760**	**412**	**959**	**814**	**387**	**188**
001-139	**I Infectious and parasitic diseases**	**98**	**18**	**29**	**27**	**13**	**11**
460-519	**VIII Diseases of the respiratory system**	**306**	**54**	**104**	**84**	**47**	**17**
460-465	Diseases of upper respiratory tract	27	9	12	5	1	-
466	Acute bronchitis and bronchiolitis	87	12	31	26	13	5
480-486	Pneumonia	129	21	45	31	24	8
740-759	**XIV Congenital anomalies**	**465**	**50**	**142**	**146**	**85**	**42**
740	Anencephalus and similar anomalies	1	1	-	-	-	-
741	Spina bifida	42	6	13	14	9	-
742	Other congenital anomalies of nervous system	45	5	11	16	8	5
745-747	Congenital anomalies of heart and circulatory system	263	25	84	85	48	21
760-779	**XV Certain conditions originating in the perinatal period**	**202**	**14**	**61**	**74**	**35**	**18**
798	Sudden death, cause unknown	1,284	228	482	349	146	79
E800-E999	**EXVII External causes of injury and poisoning**	**94**	**20**	**37**	**22**	**10**	**5**
E911	Inhalation and ingestion of food causing obstruction of respiratory tract or suffocation	30	6	11	5	7	1
E913	Accidental mechanical suffocation	11	4	3	3	1	-
	Rates						
	All causes	**4.2**	**7.2**	**5.0**	**3.6**	**3.0**	**3.5**
001-139	**I Infectious and parasitic diseases**	**0.1**	*0.3*	**0.2**	**0.1**	*0.1*	*0.2*
460-519	**VIII Diseases of the respiratory system**	**0.5**	**0.9**	**0.5**	**0.4**	**0.4**	*0.3*
460-465	Diseases of upper respiratory tract	**0.0**	*0.2*	*0.1*	*0.0*	*0.0*	-
466	Acute bronchitis and bronchiolitis	**0.1**	*0.2*	0.2	0.1	*0.1*	*0.1*
480-486	Pneumonia	**0.2**	0.4	0.2	0.1	0.2	*0.2*
740-759	**XIV Congenital anomalies**	**0.7**	**0.9**	**0.7**	**0.6**	**0.7**	**0.8**
740	Anencephalus and similar anomalies	*0.0*	*0.0*	-	-	-	-
741	Spina bifida	**0.1**	*0.1*	*0.1*	*0.1*	*0.1*	-
742	Other congenital anomalies of nervous system	**0.1**	*0.1*	*0.1*	*0.1*	*0.1*	*0.1*
745-747	Congenital anomalies of heart and circulatory system	**0.4**	0.4	0.4	0.4	0.4	0.4
760-779	**XV Certain conditions originating in the perinatal period**	**0.3**	*0.2*	**0.3**	**0.3**	**0.3**	*0.3*
798	Sudden death, cause unknown	**1.9**	4.0	2.5	1.5	1.1	1.5
E800-E999	**EXVII External causes of injury and poisoning**	**0.1**	**0.3**	**0.2**	**0.1**	*0.1*	*0.1*
E911	Inhalation and ingestion of food causing obstruction of respiratory tract or suffocation	**0.0**	*0.1*	*0.1*	*0.0*	*0.1*	*0.0*
E913	Accidental mechanical suffocation	*0.0*	*0.1*	*0.0*	*0.0*	*0.0*	-

Table 16a   Stillbirths (a), and neonatal deaths (b) - numbers: England and Wales
parity (legitimate only) by cause of death, 1986

ICD number	Cause of death			Parity of mother (legitimate only)							Illegitimate
				All	0	1	2	3	4	5 and over	
	All causes	Stillbirths	(a)	2,600	1,141	731	403	177	71	77	949
		Neonatal deaths	(b)	2,461	1,025	807	365	159	58	47	988
	Fetal mentions		(a)	1,992	859	558	341	124	53	57	723
			(b)	3,145	1,288	1,049	473	202	71	62	1,223
740-759	Congenital anomalies		(a)	209	84	51	39	16	8	11	74
			(b)	967	332	367	161	65	19	23	263
740	Anencephalus		(a)	28	8	9	6	3	1	1	13
			(b)	24	11	9	3	-	-	1	2
741	Spina bifida		(a)	15	10	3	-	2	-	-	6
			(b)	50	20	15	7	4	2	2	15
7420	Encephalocele		(a)	1	-	-	1	-	-	-	-
			(b)	19	11	5	-	1	1	1	7
742 rem	Other congenital anomalies of central nervous system		(a)	31	14	5	8	-	1	3	11
			(b)	46	13	22	6	3	1	1	19
745	Bulbus cordis anomalies and anomalies of cardiac septal closure		(a)	2	1	-	1	-	-	-	-
			(b)	93	42	22	14	6	7	2	22
746	Other congenital anomalies of heart		(a)	7	2	3	2	-	-	-	3
			(b)	179	60	78	25	10	2	4	45
747	Other congenital anomalies of circulatory system		(a)	1	1	-	-	-	-	-	-
			(b)	83	26	35	14	6	1	1	20
748	Congenital anomalies of respiratory system		(a)	5	3	1	1	-	-	-	2
			(b)	125	38	48	26	9	1	3	38
749-751	Cleft palate and lip; other congenital anomalies of upper alimentary tract and digestive system		(a)	10	2	2	4	1	-	1	2
			(b)	38	12	10	11	4	1	-	5
753	Congenital anomalies of urinary system		(a)	22	5	9	4	1	3	-	9
			(b)	78	23	31	14	9	-	1	23
754-756	Congenital musculoskeletal anomalies		(a)	28	17	5	2	3	-	1	5
			(b)	98	31	35	17	8	2	5	26
758	Chromosomal anomalies		(a)	17	6	4	2	2	1	2	4
			(b)	57	17	26	12	1	-	1	16
740-759 rem	Other and unspecified congenital anomalies		(a)	42	15	10	8	4	2	3	19
			(b)	77	28	31	12	4	1	1	25
764,765	Prematurity		(a)	129	66	33	17	6	3	4	52
			(b)	557	239	180	72	35	17	14	325
764	Slow fetal growth and fetal malnutrition		(a)	104	59	25	10	3	3	4	43
			(b)	8	4	3	1	-	-	-	4
765	Disorders relating to short gestation and unspecified low birthweight		(a)	25	7	8	7	3	-	-	9
			(b)	549	235	177	71	35	17	14	321
7650	Extreme immaturity		(a)	2	-	2	-	-	-	-	1
			(b)	394	173	129	43	26	14	9	240
7651	Other preterm infants		(a)	23	7	6	7	3	-	-	8
			(b)	155	62	48	28	9	3	5	81
767	Birth trauma		(a)	7	4	3	-	-	-	-	5
			(b)	59	29	22	4	2	1	1	28
7670	Subdural and cerebral haemorrhage		(a)	7	4	3	-	-	-	-	5
			(b)	52	24	21	4	1	1	1	25

Table 16a - *continued*

ICD number	Cause of death		Parity of mother (legitimate only)							Illegitimate
			All	0	1	2	3	4	5 and over	
768	Intrauterine hypoxia and birth asphyxia	(a) (b)	834 249	364 121	224 72	148 31	56 14	22 6	20 5	301 76
7680	Death from asphyxia or anoxia before onset of labour or at unspecified time	(a) (b)	686 -	294 -	191 -	117 -	49 -	18 -	17 -	244 -
7681	Death from asphyxia or anoxia during labour	(a) (b)	148 -	70 -	33 -	31 -	7 -	4 -	3 -	57 -
7689	Unspecified birth asphyxia in liveborn infant	(a) (b)	- 132	- 64	- 39	- 15	- 7	- 4	- 3	- 48
512,514, 516,518, 519,769, 770	Non-infectious respiratory disorders	(a) (b)	7 640	4 290	2 198	- 96	1 39	- 8	- 9	3 264
769	Respiratory distress syndrome	(a) (b)	- 337	- 157	- 107	- 44	- 20	- 3	- 6	- 138
770	Other respiratory conditions of fetus and newborn	(a) (b)	7 300	4 132	2 90	- 52	1 19	- 4	- 3	3 126
001-139, 320-326, 460-511, 513,771	Infections and infectious diseases	(a) (b)	5 139	4 64	1 47	- 15	- 10	- 2	- 1	5 60
320-322	Meningitis	(a) (b)	- 17	- 7	- 6	- 2	- 1	- 1	- -	- 9
480-486	Pneumonia	(a) (b)	- 32	- 12	- 15	- 2	- 3	- -	- -	- 15
771	Infections specific to the perinatal period	(a) (b)	5 77	4 39	1 21	- 11	- 4	- 1	- 1	5 31
766, 772-779	Other perinatal causes	(a) (b)	338 329	149 140	101 97	57 54	18 25	4 8	9 5	103 126
766	Disorders relating to long gestation and high birthweight	(a) (b)	8 3	7 2	1 1	- -	- -	- -	- -	1 -
772	Fetal and neonatal haemorrhage	(a) (b)	10 154	5 74	4 47	1 20	- 10	- 3	- -	4 72
773	Haemolytic disease of fetus or newborn, due to isoimmunization	(a) (b)	15 12	2 2	3 -	8 5	1 -	1 2	- 3	1 2
7730	due to Rh isoimmunization	(a) (b)	9 5	1 -	2 -	5 2	- -	1 1	- 2	1 1
774	Other perinatal jaundice	(a) (b)	- -	- -	- -	- -	- -	- -	- -	- 1
775	Endocrine and metabolic disturbances specific to the fetus and newborn	(a) (b)	6 3	4 1	- 2	1 -	1 -	- -	- -	- 2
7750	Syndrome of 'infant of a diabetic mother'	(a) (b)	6 -	4 -	- -	1 -	1 -	- -	- -	- -
776	Haematological disorders of fetus and newborn	(a) (b)	2 11	- 6	2 3	- 1	- -	- -	- 1	- 5
777	Perinatal disorders of digestive system	(a) (b)	- 37	- 12	- 14	- 8	- 2	- 1	- -	- 17
778	Conditions involving the integument and temperature regulation of fetus and newborn	(a) (b)	17 25	6 9	5 6	3 6	3 2	- 2	- -	3 5

Table 16a - *continued*

ICD number	Cause of death		Parity of mother (legitimate only)							Illegitimate
			All	0	1	2	3	4	5 and over	
779	Other and ill-defined conditions originating in the perinatal period	(a)	280	125	86	44	13	3	9	94
		(b)	84	34	24	14	11	-	1	22
7799	Unspecified perinatal conditions	(a)	270	125	78	43	13	2	9	93
		(b)	-	-	-	-	-	-	-	-
4275, 428, 584-586, 780-799, 800-999	Ill-defined conditions, modes of death, injury and poisoning	(a)	2	1	1	-	-	-	-	-
		(b)	102	32	30	27	8	3	2	51
798	Sudden death, cause unknown	(a)	-	-	-	-	-	-	-	-
		(b)	52	14	19	11	6	1	1	26
7980	Sudden infant death syndrome	(a)	-	-	-	-	-	-	-	-
		(b)	52	14	19	11	6	1	1	26
760-763	Maternal conditions certified as fetal	(a)	453	181	138	79	26	16	13	174
		(b)	22	8	9	4	-	1	-	13
001-E999 rem	Other fetal causes	(a)	8	2	4	1	1	-	-	6
		(b)	81	33	27	9	4	6	2	17
7996	No fetal cause	(a)	816	371	227	100	66	26	26	295
		(b)	4	3	-	-	-	1	-	1
	Maternal mentions	(a)	968	431	243	164	66	33	31	374
		(b)	649	290	198	89	40	18	14	257
642, 7600	Hypertension	(a)	192	105	41	25	11	4	6	62
		(b)	89	65	15	5	3	-	1	28
647,648, 760 rem	Other maternal conditions which may be unrelated to the present pregnancy	(a)	24	9	8	4	1	1	1	6
		(b)	15	1	5	6	2	-	1	3
761	Maternal complications in pregnancy	(a)	-	-	-	-	-	-	-	-
		(b)	1	-	1	-	-	-	-	-
762	Complications of placenta, cord and membranes	(a)	-	-	-	-	-	-	-	-
		(b)	-	-	-	-	-	-	-	-
651, 7615	Multiple pregnancy	(a)	35	12	13	7	1	1	1	9
		(b)	45	22	11	9	1	-	2	16
630-639, 643,646, 650,663, 655-658, 670-676, 761-762 rem	Other maternal complications of pregnancy, placenta, cord or membranes	(a)	239	115	52	46	14	7	5	94
		(b)	177	61	60	28	14	7	7	55
7622	Other and unspecified morphological and functional abnormalities of placenta	(a)	-	-	-	-	-	-	-	-
		(b)	-	-	-	-	-	-	-	-
7624	Prolapsed cord	(a)	-	-	-	-	-	-	-	-
		(b)	-	-	-	-	-	-	-	-
7625	Other compression of umbilical cord	(a)	-	-	-	-	-	-	-	-
		(b)	-	-	-	-	-	-	-	-
640,641, 7620, 7621	Maternal antepartum haemorrhage	(a)	351	145	86	60	32	13	15	155
		(b)	116	51	33	21	6	3	2	64
7620	Placenta praevia	(a)	-	-	-	-	-	-	-	-
		(b)	-	-	-	-	-	-	-	-

Table 16a - *continued*

ICD number	Cause of death		Parity of mother (legitimate only)							Illegitimate
			All	0	1	2	3	4	5 and over	
7621	Other forms of placental separation and haemorrhage	(a) (b)	- -	- -	- -	- -	- -	- -	- -	- -
644,645, 652-654, 659-662, 664-669, 7610, 7617,763	Complications of presentation, labour and delivery	(a) (b)	31 152	10 65	11 54	6 14	2 13	2 5	- 1	14 60
763	Other complications of labour and delivery	(a) (b)	- 1	- -	- -	- -	- 1	- -	- -	- -
001- E999 rem	Other maternal conditions	(a) (b)	96 55	35 25	32 20	16 6	5 1	5 3	3 -	34 31
7996	No maternal cause	(a) (b)	1,702 1,875	736 760	505 632	255 286	115 123	41 41	50 33	606 762
Total live births		M F P	266,517 253,156 519,673	105,507 100,079 205,586	96,791 91,748 188,539	41,744 39,716 81,460	14,074 13,546 27,620	4,784 4,568 9,352	3,617 3,499 7,116	72,335 69,010 141,345

Table 16b Stillbirths (a), and neonatal deaths (b) - rates per 1,000 total/live births: parity (legitimate only)by selected cause of death, 1986   **England and Wales**

N - list number	Cause of death			Parity of mother (legitimate only)							Illegitimate
				All	0	1	2	3	4	5 and over	
	All causes	**Stillbirth rates**	(a)	**5.0**	5.5	3.9	4.9	6.4	7.5	10.7	6.7
		Neonatal death rates	(b)	**4.7**	5.0	4.3	4.5	5.8	6.2	6.6	7.0
	Fetal mentions		(a)	**3.8**	4.2	2.9	4.2	4.5	5.6	7.9	5.1
			(b)	**6.1**	6.3	5.6	5.8	7.3	7.6	8.7	8.7
N01	Anencephalus		(a)	**0.1**	0.0	0.0	0.1	0.1	0.1	0.1	0.1
			(b)	**0.0**	0.1	0.0	0.0	-	-	0.1	0.0
N02	Spina bifida		(a)	**0.0**	0.0	0.0	-	0.1	-	-	0.0
			(b)	**0.1**	0.1	0.1	0.1	0.1	0.2	0.3	0.1
N03	Encephalocele		(a)	**0.0**	-	-	0.0	-	-	-	-
			(b)	**0.0**	0.1	0.0	-	0.0	0.1	0.1	0.0
N04	Other congenital anomalies of central nervous system		(a)	**0.1**	0.1	0.0	0.1	-	0.1	0.4	0.1
			(b)	**0.1**	0.1	0.1	0.1	0.1	0.1	0.1	0.1
N05	Congenital anomalies of circulatory system		(a)	**0.0**	0.0	0.0	0.0	-	-	-	0.0
			(b)	**0.7**	0.6	0.7	0.7	0.8	1.1	1.0	0.6
N06	Other congenital anomalies		(a)	**0.2**	0.2	0.2	0.3	0.4	0.6	1.0	0.3
			(b)	**0.9**	0.7	1.0	1.1	1.3	0.5	1.5	0.9
N07	Prematurity		(a)	**0.2**	0.3	0.2	0.2	0.2	0.3	0.6	0.4
			(b)	**1.1**	1.2	1.0	0.9	1.3	1.8	2.0	2.3
N08	Birth trauma		(a)	**0.0**	0.0	0.0	-	-	-	-	0.0
			(b)	**0.1**	0.1	0.1	0.0	0.1	0.1	0.1	0.2
N09	Birth asphyxia		(a)	**1.6**	1.8	1.2	1.8	2.0	2.3	2.8	2.1
			(b)	**0.5**	0.6	0.4	0.4	0.5	0.6	0.7	0.5
N10	Non-infectious respiratory disorders		(a)	**0.0**	0.0	0.0	-	0.0	-	-	0.0
			(b)	**1.2**	1.4	1.1	1.2	1.4	0.9	1.3	1.9
N11	Infections and infectious diseases		(a)	**0.0**	0.0	0.0	-	-	-	-	0.0
			(b)	**0.3**	0.3	0.2	0.2	0.4	0.2	0.1	0.4
N12	Other perinatal causes		(a)	**0.6**	0.7	0.5	0.7	0.6	0.4	1.3	0.7
			(b)	**0.6**	0.7	0.5	0.7	0.9	0.9	0.7	0.9
N13	Ill-defined conditions, modes of death, injury and poisoning		(a)	**0.0**	0.0	0.0	-	-	-	-	-
			(b)	**0.2**	0.2	0.2	0.3	0.3	0.3	0.3	0.4
N14	Maternal conditions classified as fetal		(a)	**0.9**	0.9	0.7	1.0	0.9	1.7	1.8	1.2
			(b)	**0.0**	0.0	0.0	0.0	-	0.1	-	0.1
N15	Other fetal causes		(a)	**0.0**	0.0	0.0	0.0	0.0	-	-	0.0
			(b)	**0.2**	0.2	0.1	0.1	0.1	0.6	0.3	0.1
N16	No fetal cause		(a)	**1.6**	1.8	1.2	1.2	2.4	2.8	3.6	2.1
			(b)	**0.0**	0.0	-	-	-	0.1	-	0.0
	Maternal mentions		(a)	**1.9**	2.1	1.3	2.0	2.4	3.5	4.3	2.6
			(b)	**1.2**	1.4	1.1	1.1	1.4	1.9	2.0	1.8
N17	Hypertension		(a)	**0.4**	0.5	0.2	0.3	0.4	0.4	0.8	0.4
			(b)	**0.2**	0.3	0.1	0.1	0.1	-	0.1	0.2
N18	Other maternal conditions which may be unrelated to the present pregnancy		(a)	**0.0**	0.0	0.0	0.0	0.0	0.1	0.1	0.0
			(b)	**0.0**	0.0	0.0	0.1	0.1	-	0.1	0.0
N19	Multiple pregnancy		(a)	**0.1**	0.1	0.1	0.1	0.0	0.1	0.1	0.1
			(b)	**0.1**	0.1	0.1	0.1	0.0	-	0.3	0.1
N20	Other maternal complications related to pregnancy, placenta, cord or membranes		(a)	**0.5**	0.6	0.3	0.6	0.5	0.7	0.7	0.7
			(b)	**0.3**	0.3	0.3	0.3	0.5	0.7	1.0	0.4

Table 16b - *continued*

N - list number	Cause of death		Parity of mother (legitimate only)							Illegitimate
			All	0	1	2	3	4	5 and over	
N21	Maternal antepartum	(a)	0.7	0.7	0.5	0.7	1.2	*1.4*	*2.1*	1.1
	haemorrhage	(b)	0.2	0.2	0.2	0.3	*0.2*	*0.3*	*0.3*	0.5
N22	Complications of presentation,	(a)	0.1	*0.0*	*0.1*	*0.1*	*0.1*	0.2	-	*0.1*
	labour and delivery	(b)	0.3	0.3	0.3	*0.2*	*0.5*	*0.5*	*0.1*	0.4
N23	Other maternal conditions	(a)	0.2	0.2	0.2	*0.2*	*0.2*	*0.5*	*0.4*	0.2
		(b)	0.1	0.1	0.1	*0.1*	*0.0*	*0.3*	-	0.2
N24	No maternal cause	(a)	3.3	3.6	2.7	3.1	4.1	4.4	7.0	4.3
		(b)	3.6	3.7	3.4	3.5	4.5	4.4	4.6	5.4

Table 17 Postneonatal deaths - numbers and rates per 1,000 live births:
parity (legitimate only) by selected cause of death, 1986
England and Wales

ICD number	Cause of death	All	Parity of mother (legitimate only)					Illegit - imate
			All	0	1	2	3 and over	
	Numbers							
	All causes	**2,760**	**1,901**	**538**	**725**	**405**	**233**	**859**
001-139	**I Infectious and parasitic diseases**	**98**	**63**	**15**	**20**	**20**	**8**	**35**
460-519	**VIII Diseases of the respiratory system**	**306**	**214**	**42**	**89**	**52**	**31**	**92**
460-465	Diseases of upper respiratory tract	27	17	4	7	5	1	10
466	Acute bronchitis and bronchiolitis	87	66	10	28	22	6	21
480-486	Pneumonia	129	85	18	34	17	16	44
740-759	**XIV Congenital anomalies**	**465**	**354**	**114**	**134**	**62**	**44**	**111**
740	Anencephalus and similar anomalies	1	-	-	-	-	-	1
741	Spina bifida	42	38	13	12	10	3	4
742	Other congenital anomalies of nervous system	45	34	9	12	7	6	11
745-747	Congenital anomalies of heart and circulatory system	263	197	66	78	31	22	66
760-779	**XV Certain conditions originating in the perinatal period**	**202**	**143**	**63**	**44**	**23**	**13**	**59**
798	Sudden death, cause unknown	1,284	833	212	337	199	85	451
E800-E999	**EXVII External causes of injury and poisoning**	**94**	**59**	**24**	**22**	**2**	**11**	**35**
E911	Inhalation and ingestion of food causing obstruction of respiratory tract or suffocation	30	22	7	11	-	4	8
E913	Accidental mechanical suffocation	11	4	1	2	-	1	7
	Rates							
	All causes	**4.2**	**3.7**	**2.6**	**3.8**	**5.0**	**5.3**	**6.1**
001-139	**I Infectious and parasitic diseases**	**0.1**	**0.1**	*0.1*	**0.1**	**0.2**	*0.2*	**0.2**
460-519	**VIII Diseases of the respiratory system**	**0.5**	**0.4**	**0.2**	**0.5**	**0.6**	**0.7**	**0.7**
460-465	Diseases of upper respiratory tract	0.0	*0.0*	*0.0*	*0.0*	*0.1*	*0.0*	*0.1*
466	Acute bronchitis and bronchiolitis	0.1	0.1	*0.0*	0.1	0.3	*0.1*	0.1
480-486	Pneumonia	0.2	0.2	*0.1*	0.2	*0.2*	*0.4*	0.3
740-759	**XIV Congenital anomalies**	**0.7**	**0.7**	**0.6**	**0.7**	**0.8**	**1.0**	**0.8**
740	Anencephalus and similar anomalies	*0.0*	-	-	-	-	-	*0.0*
741	Spina bifida	0.1	0.1	*0.1*	0.1	*0.1*	*0.1*	0.0
742	Other congenital anomalies of nervous system	0.1	0.1	*0.0*	*0.1*	*0.1*	*0.1*	*0.1*
745-747	Congenital anomalies of heart and circulatory system	0.4	0.4	0.3	0.4	0.4	0.5	0.5
760-779	**XV Certain conditions originating in the perinatal period**	**0.3**	**0.3**	**0.3**	**0.2**	**0.3**	*0.3*	**0.4**
798	Sudden death, cause unknown	1.9	1.6	1.0	1.8	2.4	1.9	3.2
E800-E999	**EXVII External causes of injury and poisoning**	**0.1**	**0.1**	**0.1**	**0.1**	*0.0*	**0.2**	**0.2**
E911	Inhalation and ingestion of food causing obstruction of respiratory tract or suffocation	**0.0**	0.0	*0.0*	*0.1*	-	*0.1*	*0.1*
E913	Accidental mechanical suffocation	*0.0*	*0.0*	*0.0*	*0.0*	-	*0.0*	*0.0*

Table 18a Stillbirths (a), and neonatal deaths (b) - numbers: social class (legitimate only) by cause of death, 1986 **England and Wales**

ICD number	Cause of death		Social class (legitimate only)									Illegitimate
			All	I - V	I	II	IIIN	IIIM	IV	V	Others	
	All causes											
	Stillbirths	(a)	2,600	2,439	150	478	267	939	419	186	161	949
	Neonatal deaths	(b)	2,461	2,289	167	485	237	841	391	168	172	988
	Fetal mentions	(a)	1,992	1,861	106	376	206	720	308	145	131	723
		(b)	3,145	2,931	205	622	310	1,087	495	212	214	1,223
740-759	Congenital anomalies	(a)	209	190	8	33	25	63	40	21	19	74
		(b)	967	900	69	186	96	333	153	63	67	263
740	Anencephalus	(a)	28	26	3	3	2	13	3	2	2	13
		(b)	24	20	3	2	1	10	2	2	4	2
741	Spina bifida	(a)	15	13	3	-	3	2	5	-	2	6
		(b)	50	44	3	10	5	18	7	1	6	15
7420	Encephalocele	(a)	1	1	-	1	-	-	-	-	-	-
		(b)	19	16	2	-	1	7	3	3	3	7
742 rem	Other congenital anomalies of central nervous system	(a)	31	31	2	7	4	9	5	4	-	11
		(b)	46	44	5	7	7	16	7	2	2	19
745	Bulbus cordis anomalies and anomalies of cardiac septal closure	(a)	2	2	-	1	-	-	1	-	-	-
		(b)	93	92	7	29	3	37	10	6	1	22
746	Other congenital anomalies of heart	(a)	7	5	-	1	1	1	-	2	2	3
		(b)	179	171	13	34	19	63	36	6	8	45
747	Other congenital anomalies of circulatory system	(a)	1	1	-	-	-	1	-	-	-	-
		(b)	83	77	7	14	8	31	13	4	6	20
748	Congenital anomalies of respiratory system	(a)	5	4	-	2	-	1	-	1	1	2
		(b)	125	116	8	26	16	42	15	9	9	38
749-751	Cleft palate and lip; other congenital anomalies of upper alimentary tract and digestive system	(a)	10	10	-	4	-	1	3	2	-	2
		(b)	38	38	2	10	4	14	2	6	-	
753	Congenital anomalies of urinary system	(a)	22	19	-	3	4	6	3	3	3	9
		(b)	78	65	4	6	14	21	14	6	13	23
754-756	Congenital musculoskeletal anomalies	(a)	28	24	-	1	7	8	6	2	4	5
		(b)	98	92	6	24	7	29	16	10	6	26
758	Chromosomal anomalies	(a)	17	17	-	4	1	6	5	1	-	4
		(b)	57	54	5	8	4	20	12	5	3	16
740-759 rem	Other and unspecified congenital anomalies	(a)	42	37	-	6	3	15	9	4	5	19
		(b)	77	71	4	16	7	25	16	3	6	25
764,765	Prematurity	(a)	129	121	7	26	16	39	26	7	8	52
		(b)	557	520	36	119	40	207	75	43	37	325
764	Slow fetal growth and fetal malnutrition	(a)	104	98	5	22	14	32	19	6	6	43
		(b)	8	8	1	1	-	4	2	-	-	4

Table 18a - *continued*

ICD number	Cause of death		Social class (legitimate only)									Illegitimate
			All	I - V	I	II	IIIN	IIIM	IV	V	Others	
765	Disorders relating to short gestation and unspecified low birthweight	(a)	25	23	2	4	2	7	7	1	2	9
		(b)	549	512	35	118	40	203	73	43	37	321
7650	Extreme immaturity	(a)	2	2	1	-	-	1	-	-	-	1
		(b)	394	366	20	90	29	144	51	32	28	240
7651	Other preterm infants	(a)	23	21	1	4	2	6	7	1	2	8
		(b)	155	146	15	28	11	59	22	11	9	81
767	Birth trauma	(a)	7	7	-	2	1	2	1	1	-	5
		(b)	59	54	5	7	3	26	7	6	5	28
7670	Subdural and cerebral haemorrhage	(a)	7	7	-	2	1	2	1	1	-	5
		(b)	52	49	5	6	3	22	7	6	3	25
768	Intrauterine hypoxia and birth asphyxia	(a)	834	772	47	151	82	300	131	61	62	301
		(b)	249	231	15	49	34	83	37	13	18	76
7680	Death from asphyxia or anoxia before onset of labour or at unspecified time	(a)	686	634	37	126	68	249	104	50	52	244
		(b)	.	-	-	-	-	-	-	-	-	-
7681	Death from asphyxia or anoxia during labour	(a)	148	138	10	25	14	51	27	11	10	57
		(b)	.	-	-	-	-	-	-	-	-	-
7689	Unspecified birth asphyxia in liveborn infant	(a)	.	-	-	-	-	-	-	-	-	-
		(b)	132	123	5	33	18	39	19	9	9	48
512,514, 516,518, 519,769, 770	Non-infectious respiratory disorders	(a)	7	7	-	2	-	3	1	1	-	3
		(b)	640	609	44	129	65	214	113	44	31	264
769	Respiratory distress syndrome	(a)	.	-	-	-	-	-	-	-	-	-
		(b)	337	319	23	75	26	104	63	28	18	138
770	Other respiratory conditions of fetus and newborn	(a)	7	7	-	2	-	3	1	1	-	3
		(b)	300	287	21	54	38	110	49	15	13	126
001-139, 320-326, 460-511, 513,771	Infections and infectious diseases	(a)	5	5	1	2	-	1	1	-	-	5
		(b)	139	131	9	28	19	45	20	10	8	60
320-322	Meningitis	(a)	.	-	-	-	-	-	-	-	-	-
		(b)	17	17	1	3	2	7	4	-	-	9
480-486	Pneumonia	(a)	.	-	-	-	-	-	-	-	-	-
		(b)	32	29	3	7	3	10	2	4	3	15
771	Infections specific to the perinatal period	(a)	5	5	1	2	-	1	1	-	-	5
		(b)	77	72	4	16	12	23	12	5	5	31
766, 772-779	Other perinatal causes	(a)	338	321	15	57	40	132	50	27	17	103
		(b)	329	306	15	63	35	116	52	25	23	126
766	Disorders relating to long gestation and high birthweight	(a)	8	8	-	1	1	3	3	-	-	1
		(b)	3	3	-	1	-	1	1	-	-	-
772	Fetal and neonatal haemorrhage	(a)	10	10	-	3	1	2	1	3	-	4
		(b)	154	146	5	32	18	63	19	9	8	72
773	Haemolytic disease of fetus or newborn, due to isoimmunization	(a)	15	14	-	2	1	8	2	1	1	1
		(b)	12	12	-	-	-	5	2	5	-	2

Table 18a - *continued*

ICD number	Cause of death		All	I - V	I	II	IIIN	IIIM	IV	V	Others	Illegitimate
7730	Due to Rh isoimmunization	(a)	9	8	-	2	1	4	1	-	1	1
		(b)	5	5	-	-	-	2	-	3	-	1
774	Other perinatal jaundice	(a)	·	-	-	-	-	-	-	-	-	-
		(b)	·	-	-	-	-	-	-	-	-	1
775	Endocrine and metabolic disturbances specific to the fetus and newborn	(a)	6	6	-	1	-	3	2	-	-	-
		(b)	3	3	-	2	-	-	1	-	-	2
7750	Syndrome of 'infant of a diabetic mother'	(a)	6	6	-	1	-	3	2	-	-	-
		(b)	·	-	-	-	-	-	-	-	-	-
776	Haematological disorders of fetus and newborn	(a)	2	2	-	-	-	1	1	-	-	-
		(b)	11	10	2	2	-	4	2	-	1	5
777	Perinatal disorders of digestive system	(a)	·	-	-	-	-	-	-	-	-	-
		(b)	37	35	2	6	7	11	5	4	2	17
778	Conditions involving the integument and temperature regulation of fetus and newborn	(a)	17	17	4	3	3	5	1	1	-	3
		(b)	25	18	2	3	2	4	5	2	7	5
779	Other and ill-defined conditions originating in the perinatal period	(a)	280	264	11	47	34	110	40	22	16	94
		(b)	84	79	4	17	8	28	17	5	5	22
7799	Unspecified perinatal conditions	(a)	270	255	11	45	34	106	37	22	15	93
		(b)	·	-	-	-	-	-	-	-	-	-
4275, 428, 584-586, 780-799, 800-999	Ill-defined conditions, modes of death, injury and poisoning	(a)	2	2	-	1	-	-	1	-	-	-
		(b)	102	90	2	22	10	30	21	5	12	51
798	Sudden death, cause unknown	(a)	·	-	-	-	-	-	-	-	-	-
		(b)	52	48	1	13	1	13	15	5	4	26
7980	Sudden infant death syndrome	(a)	·	-	-	-	-	-	-	-	-	-
		(b)	52	48	1	13	1	13	15	5	4	26
760-763	Maternal conditions certified as fetal	(a)	453	428	28	100	42	175	57	26	25	174
		(b)	22	20	1	5	3	7	4	-	2	13
001-E999 rem	Other fetal causes	(a)	8	8	-	2	-	5	-	1	-	6
		(b)	81	70	9	14	5	26	13	3	11	17
7996	No fetal cause	(a)	816	771	50	146	81	300	131	63	45	295
		(b)	4	3	-	-	-	2	1	-	1	1
	Maternal mentions	(a)	968	908	47	162	86	374	166	73	60	374
		(b)	649	609	34	134	67	240	85	49	40	257
642, 7600	Hypertension	(a)	192	178	12	30	13	75	30	18	14	62
		(b)	89	82	4	19	11	31	15	2	7	28
647,648, 760 rem	Other maternal conditions which may be unrelated to the present pregnancy	(a)	24	22	1	-	3	9	6	3	2	6
		(b)	15	14	1	-	2	9	2	-	1	3

Table 18a - *continued*

ICD number	Cause of death		Social class (legitimate only)									Illegit- imate
			All	I - V	I	II	IIIN	IIIM	IV	V	Others	
761	Maternal complications in pregnancy	(a)	·	-	-	-	-	-	-	-	-	-
		(b)	1	1	-	-	-	1	-	-	-	-
762	Complications of placenta, cord and membranes	(a)	·	-	-	-	-	-	-	-	-	-
		(b)	·	-	-	-	-	-	-	-	-	-
651, 7615	Multiple pregnancy	(a)	35	33	2	2	6	12	9	2	2	9
		(b)	45	44	2	11	6	19	4	2	1	16
630-639, 643,646, 650,663, 655-658, 670-676, 761-762 rem	Other maternal complications of pregnancy, placenta, cord or membranes	(a)	239	227	9	52	23	87	41	15	12	94
		(b)	177	166	8	39	16	57	25	21	11	55
7622	Other and unspecified morphological and functional abnormalities of placenta	(a)	·	-	-	-	-	-	-	-	-	-
		(b)	·	-	-	-	-	-	-	-	-	-
7624	Prolapsed cord	(a)	·	-	-	-	-	-	-	-	-	-
		(b)	·	-	-	-	-	-	-	-	-	-
7625	Other compression of umbilical cord	(a)	·	-	-	-	-	-	-	-	-	-
		(b)	·	-	-	-	-	-	-	-	-	-
640,641, 7620, 7621	Maternal antepartum haemorrhage	(a)	351	330	16	55	26	148	61	24	21	155
		(b)	116	108	5	29	13	37	13	11	8	64
7620	Placenta praevia	(a)	·	-	-	-	-	-	-	-	-	-
		(b)	·	-	-	-	-	-	-	-	-	-
7621	Other forms of placental separation and haemorrhage	(a)	·	-	-	-	-	-	-	-	-	-
		(b)	·	-	-	-	-	-	-	-	-	-
644,645, 652-654, 659-662, 664-669, 7610, 7617,763	Complications of presentation, labour and delivery	(a)	31	27	2	8	6	9	1	1	4	14
		(b)	152	142	7	28	14	64	19	10	10	60
763	Other complications of labour and delivery	(a)	·	-	-	-	-	-	-	-	-	-
		(b)	1	1	-	-	-	-	1	-	-	-
001- E999 rem	Other maternal conditions	(a)	96	91	5	15	9	34	18	10	5	34
		(b)	55	53	7	8	5	23	7	3	2	31
7996	No maternal cause	(a)	1,702	1,598	108	328	189	592	262	119	104	606
		(b)	1,875	1,741	137	368	173	629	312	122	134	762
Total live births		M	266,839	254,920	20,890	61,450	28,780	92,020	37,340	14,440	11,920	72,340
		F	252,834	240,960	19,920	57,850	26,440	87,470	35,550	13,730	11,880	69,010
		P	519,673	495,880	40,810	119,300	55,220	179,500	72,890	28,170	23,790	141,340

Table 18b Stillbirths (a), and neonatal deaths (b) - rates per 1,000 total/live births: England and Wales
social class (legitimate only) by selected cause of death, 1986

N-list number	Cause of death	Social class (legitimate only)									Illegitimate
		All	I - V	I	II	IIIN	IIIM	IV	V	Others	
	All causes										
	Stillbirth rates	(a) 5.0	4.9	3.7	4.0	4.8	5.2	5.7	6.6	6.7	6.7
	Neonatal death rates	(b) 4.7	4.6	4.1	4.1	4.3	4.7	5.4	6.0	7.2	7.0
	Fetal mentions	(a) 3.8	3.7	2.6	3.1	3.7	4.0	4.2	5.1	5.5	5.1
		(b) 6.1	5.9	5.0	5.2	5.6	6.1	6.8	7.5	9.0	8.7
N01	Anencephalus	(a) 0.1	0.1	0.1	0.0	0.0	0.1	0.0	0.1	0.1	0.1
		(b) 0.0	0.0	0.1	0.0	0.0	0.1	0.0	0.1	0.2	0.0
N02	Spina bifida	(a) 0.0	0.0	0.1	-	0.1	0.0	0.1	-	0.1	0.0
		(b) 0.1	0.1	0.1	0.1	0.1	0.1	0.1	0.0	0.3	0.1
N03	Encephalocele	(a) 0.0	0.0	-	0.0	-	-	-	-	-	-
		(b) 0.0	0.0	0.0	-	0.0	0.0	0.0	0.1	0.1	0.0
N04	Other congenital anomalies of central nervous system	(a) 0.1	0.1	0.0	0.1	0.1	0.0	0.1	0.1	-	0.1
		(b) 0.1	0.1	0.1	0.1	0.1	0.1	0.1	0.1	0.1	0.1
N05	Congenital anomalies of circulatory system	(a) 0.0	0.0	-	0.0	0.0	0.0	0.0	0.1	0.1	0.0
		(b) 0.7	0.7	0.7	0.6	0.5	0.7	0.8	0.6	0.6	0.6
N06	Other congenital anomalies	(a) 0.2	0.2	-	0.2	0.3	0.2	0.4	0.5	0.5	0.3
		(b) 0.9	0.9	0.7	0.8	0.9	0.8	1.0	1.4	1.6	0.9
N07	Prematurity	(a) 0.2	0.2	0.2	0.2	0.3	0.2	0.4	0.2	0.3	0.4
		(b) 1.1	1.0	0.9	1.0	0.7	1.2	1.0	1.5	1.6	2.3
N08	Birth trauma	(a) 0.0	0.0	-	0.0	0.0	0.0	0.0	0.0	-	0.0
		(b) 0.1	0.1	0.1	0.1	0.1	0.1	0.1	0.2	0.2	0.2
N09	Birth asphyxia	(a) 1.6	1.5	1.1	1.3	1.5	1.7	1.8	2.2	2.6	2.1
		(b) 0.5	0.5	0.4	0.4	0.6	0.5	0.5	0.5	0.8	0.5
N10	Non-infectious respiratory disorders	(a) 0.0	0.0	-	0.0	-	0.0	0.0	0.0	-	0.0
		(b) 1.2	1.2	1.1	1.1	1.2	1.2	1.6	1.6	1.3	1.9
N11	Infections and infectious diseases	(a) 0.0	0.0	0.0	0.0	-	0.0	0.0	-	-	0.0
		(b) 0.3	0.3	0.2	0.2	0.3	0.3	0.3	0.4	0.3	0.4
N12	Other perinatal causes	(a) 0.6	0.6	0.4	0.5	0.7	0.7	0.7	1.0	0.7	0.7
		(b) 0.6	0.6	0.4	0.5	0.6	0.6	0.7	0.9	1.0	0.9
N13	Ill-defined conditions, modes of death, injury and poisoning	(a) 0.0	0.0	-	0.0	-	-	0.0	-	-	-
		(b) 0.2	0.2	0.0	0.2	0.2	0.2	0.3	0.2	0.5	0.4
N14	Maternal conditions classified as fetal	(a) 0.9	0.9	0.7	0.8	0.8	1.0	0.8	0.9	1.0	1.2
		(b) 0.0	0.0	0.0	0.0	0.1	0.0	0.1	-	0.1	0.1
N15	Other fetal causes	(a) 0.0	0.0	-	0.0	-	0.0	-	0.0	-	0.0
		(b) 0.2	0.1	0.2	0.1	0.1	0.1	0.2	0.1	0.5	0.1
N16	No fetal cause	(a) 1.6	1.5	1.2	1.2	1.5	1.7	1.8	2.2	1.9	2.1
		(b) 0.0	0.0	-	-	-	0.0	0.0	-	0.0	0.0
	Maternal mentions	(a) 1.9	1.8	1.1	1.4	1.5	2.1	2.3	2.6	2.5	2.6
		(b) 1.2	1.2	0.8	1.1	1.2	1.3	1.2	1.7	1.7	1.8
N17	Hypertension	(a) 0.4	0.4	0.3	0.3	0.2	0.4	0.4	0.6	0.6	0.4
		(b) 0.2	0.2	0.1	0.2	0.2	0.2	0.2	0.1	0.3	0.2
N18	Other maternal conditions which may be unrelated to the present pregnancy	(a) 0.0	0.0	0.0	-	0.1	0.0	0.1	0.1	0.1	0.0
		(b) 0.0	0.0	0.0	-	0.0	0.1	0.0	-	0.0	0.0

Table 18b - *continued*

N-list number	Cause of death		Social class (legitimate only)									Illegit-imate
			All	I - V	I	II	IIIN	IIIM	IV	V	Others	
N19	Multiple pregnancy	(a)	0.1	0.1	0.0	0.0	0.1	0.1	0.1	0.1	0.1	0.1
		(b)	0.1	0.1	0.0	0.1	0.1	0.1	0.1	0.1	0.0	0.1
N20	Other maternal complications related to pregnancy, placenta, cord or membranes	(a)	0.5	0.5	0.2	0.4	0.4	0.5	0.6	0.5	0.5	0.7
		(b)	0.3	0.3	0.2	0.3	0.3	0.3	0.3	0.7	0.5	0.4
N21	Maternal antepartum haemorrhage	(a)	0.7	0.7	0.4	0.5	0.5	0.8	0.8	0.8	0.9	1.1
		(b)	0.2	0.2	0.1	0.2	0.2	0.2	0.2	0.4	0.3	0.5
N22	Complications of presentation, labour and delivery	(a)	0.1	0.1	0.0	0.1	0.1	0.0	0.0	0.0	0.2	0.1
		(b)	0.3	0.3	0.2	0.2	0.3	0.4	0.3	0.4	0.4	0.4
N23	Other maternal conditions	(a)	0.2	0.2	0.1	0.1	0.2	0.2	0.2	0.4	0.2	0.2
		(b)	0.1	0.1	0.2	0.1	0.1	0.1	0.1	0.1	0.1	0.2
N24	No maternal cause	(a)	3.3	3.2	2.6	2.7	3.4	3.3	3.6	4.2	4.3	4.3
		(b)	3.6	3.5	3.4	3.1	3.1	3.5	4.3	4.3	5.6	5.4

Table 19 Postneonatal deaths - numbers and rates per 1,000 live births: **England and Wales**
social class (legitimate only) selected cause of death, 1986

ICD number	Cause of death	Social class (legitimate only)									Illegit-imate
		All	I - V	I	II	IIIN	IIIM	IV	V	Others	
	Numbers										
	All causes	**1,901**	**1,737**	**109**	**353**	**168**	**616**	**344**	**147**	**164**	**859**
001-139	**I Infectious and parasitic diseases**	63	60	3	11	1	23	13	9	3	35
460-519	**VIII Diseases of the respiratory system**	214	193	8	32	12	85	36	20	21	92
460-465	Diseases of upper respiratory tract	17	16	1	1	2	7	5	-	1	10
466	Acute bronchitis and bronchiolitis	66	61	3	11	4	27	10	6	5	21
480-486	Pneumonia	85	78	1	16	2	34	16	9	7	44
740-759	**XIV Congenital anomalies**	354	334	22	78	32	115	67	20	20	111
740	Anencephalus and similar anomalies	-	-	-	-	-	-	-	-	-	1
741	Spina bifida	38	37	3	4	5	17	1	7	1	4
742	Other congenital anomalies of nervous system	34	33	1	12	4	6	10	-	1	11
745-747	Congenital anomalies of heart and circulatory system	197	184	13	46	15	65	37	8	13	66
760-779	**XV Certain conditions originating in the perinatal period**	143	137	6	26	22	52	26	5	6	59
798	Sudden death, cause unknown	833	755	57	154	69	261	152	62	78	451
E800-E999	**EXVII External causes of injury and poisoning**	59	46	2	11	7	12	8	6	13	35
E911	Inhalation of food causing obstruction of respiratory tract or suffocation	22	20	1	5	2	8	2	2	2	8
E913	Accidental mechanical suffocation	4	3	-	2	-	-	1	-	1	7
	Rates										
	All causes	**3.7**	**3.5**	**2.7**	**3.0**	**3.0**	**3.4**	**4.7**	**5.2**	**6.9**	**6.1**
001-139	**I Infectious and parasitic diseases**	0.1	0.1	*0.1*	*0.1*	0.0	0.1	*0.2*	*0.3*	*0.1*	0.2
460-519	**VIII Diseases of the respiratory system**	0.4	0.4	*0.2*	*0.3*	*0.2*	0.5	*0.5*	*0.7*	*0.9*	0.7
460-465	Diseases of upper respiratory tract	*0.0*	*0.0*	0.0	0.0	0.0	0.0	0.1	-	0.0	0.1
466	Acute bronchitis and bronchiolitis	0.1	0.1	*0.1*	0.1	*0.1*	0.2	*0.1*	0.2	0.2	0.1
480-486	Pneumonia	0.2	0.2	0.0	0.1	0.0	0.2	0.2	0.3	0.3	0.3
740-759	**XIV Congenital anomalies**	0.7	0.7	0.5	0.7	0.6	0.6	0.9	0.7	0.8	0.8
740	Anencephalus and similar anomalies	-	-	-	-	-	-	-	-	-	0.0
741	Spina bifida	0.1	0.1	*0.1*	0.0	*0.1*	*0.1*	0.0	0.2	0.0	0.0
742	Other congenital anomalies of nervous system	0.1	0.1	0.0	0.1	0.1	0.0	0.1	-	0.0	0.1
745-747	Congenital anomalies of heart and circulatory system	0.4	0.4	*0.3*	0.4	*0.3*	0.4	0.5	*0.3*	0.5	0.5
760-779	**XV Certain conditions originating in the perinatal period**	0.3	0.3	*0.1*	0.2	0.4	0.3	0.4	0.2	*0.3*	0.4
798	Sudden death, cause unknown	1.6	1.5	1.4	1.3	1.2	1.5	2.1	2.2	3.3	3.2
E800-E999	**EXVII External causes of injury and poisoning**	0.1	0.1	*0.0*	*0.1*	*0.1*	*0.1*	*0.1*	0.2	0.5	0.2
E911	Inhalation of food causing obstruction of respiratory tract or suffocation	0.0	0.0	*0.0*	0.0	0.0	0.0	0.0	0.1	0.1	0.1
E913	Accidental mechanical suffocation	*0.0*	*0.0*	-	0.0	-	-	0.0	-	0.0	0.0

Table 20 Stillbirths, neonatal deaths, postneonatal deaths and live births - numbers: **England and Wales**
number of previous stillbirths (legitimate only) by parity, 1986

	Parity (previous live and stillbirths of all marriages)	Number of previous stillbirths (legitimate only)					
		Total	0	1	2	3	4-9
Stillbirths	Total	2,600	2,496	94	10	.	.
	0	1,141	1,141	-	-	-	-
	1	731	706	25	-	-	-
	2	403	382	21	-	-	-
	3	177	149	24	4	-	-
	4	71	56	13	2	-	-
	5-9	74	59	11	4	-	-
	10 and over	3	3	-	-	-	-
Early neonatal deaths	Total	1,991	1,938	46	7	.	.
	0	830	830	-	-	-	-
	1	648	632	16	-	-	-
	2	294	281	13	-	-	-
	3	135	122	10	3	-	-
	4	43	38	4	1	-	-
	5-9	40	34	3	3	-	-
	10 and over	1	1	-	-	-	-
Late neonatal deaths	Total	470	458	12	.	.	.
	0	195	195	-	-	-	-
	1	159	156	3	-	-	-
	2	71	68	3	-	-	-
	3	24	22	2	-	-	-
	4	15	12	3	-	-	-
	5-9	6	5	1	-	-	-
	10 and over	.	-	-	-	-	-
Postneonatal deaths	Total	1,901	1,876	25	.	.	.
	0	538	538	-	-	-	-
	1	725	717	8	-	-	-
	2	405	399	6	-	-	-
	3	141	135	6	-	-	-
	4	51	51	-	-	-	-
	5-9	40	35	5	-	-	-
	10 and over	1	1	-	-	-	-
Live births	Total	519,673	513,964	5,400	273	24	12
	0	205,586	205,586	-	-	-	-
	1	188,539	187,220	1,319	-	-	-
	2	81,460	79,577	1,848	35	-	-
	3	27,620	26,322	1,192	105	1	-
	4	9,352	8,713	563	65	10	1
	5-9	6,964	6,415	464	65	12	8
	10 and over	152	131	14	3	1	3

Table 21   Stillbirths - numbers: **England and Wales**
duration of pregnancy by main fetal and main maternal causes of death, 1986

ICD number	Cause of death		Total	28-29	30-31	32-33	34-35	36-37	38-39	40	41-42	43 and over	Not stated
	All causes	P	3,549	395	416	444	452	556	567	335	202	13	169
		M	1,904	210	236	233	255	322	281	181	97	5	84
		F	1,645	185	180	211	197	234	286	154	105	8	85
	Fetal mentions	P	2,715	291	312	340	355	415	419	261	161	13	148
		M	1,457	158	168	176	203	244	212	135	77	7	77
		F	1,258	133	144	164	152	171	207	126	84	6	71
740-759	Congenital anomalies	P	283	33	40	42	42	46	39	11	9	2	19
		M	146	12	21	21	19	27	21	7	5	-	13
		F	137	21	19	21	23	19	18	4	4	2	6
740	Anencephalus	P	41	5	7	7	8	7	3	1	2	-	1
		M	15	1	-	3	4	5	-	1	1	-	-
		F	26	4	7	4	4	2	3	-	1	-	1
741	Spina bifida	P	21	2	2	3	-	2	5	2	3	-	2
		M	7	-	-	2	-	1	1	1	1	-	1
		F	14	2	2	1	-	1	4	1	2	-	1
7420	Encephalocele	P	1	1	-	-	-	-	-	-	-	-	-
		M	-	-	-	-	-	-	-	-	-	-	-
		F	1	1	-	-	-	-	-	-	-	-	-
742 rem	Other congenital anomalies of central nervous system	P	42	3	5	2	8	4	8	2	3	-	7
		M	23	2	4	-	2	3	4	1	2	-	5
		F	19	1	1	2	6	1	4	1	1	-	2
745	Bulbus cordis anomalies and anomalies of cardiac septal closure	P	2	-	-	1	-	-	-	-	-	1	-
		M	1	-	-	1	-	-	-	-	-	-	-
		F	1	-	-	-	-	-	-	-	-	1	-
746	Other congenital anomalies of heart	P	10	4	-	3	-	1	2	-	-	-	-
		M	3	-	-	2	-	-	1	-	-	-	-
		F	7	4	-	1	-	1	1	-	-	-	-
747	Other congenital anomalies of circulatory system	P	1	-	-	-	-	1	-	-	-	-	-
		M	1	-	-	-	-	1	-	-	-	-	-
		F	-	-	-	-	-	-	-	-	-	-	-
748	Congenital anomalies of respiratory system	P	7	1	-	-	-	1	2	1	-	1	1
		M	5	1	-	-	-	1	1	1	-	-	1
		F	2	-	-	-	-	-	1	-	-	1	-
749-751	Cleft palate and lip; other congenital anomalies of upper alimentary tract and digestive system	P	12	-	1	3	4	2	1	1	-	-	-
		M	3	-	-	1	1	-	-	1	-	-	-
		F	9	-	1	2	3	2	1	-	-	-	-
753	Congenital anomalies of urinary system	P	31	2	8	9	4	3	2	-	1	-	2
		M	23	1	7	6	2	3	2	-	1	-	1
		F	8	1	1	3	2	-	-	-	-	-	1
754-756	Congenital musculoskeletal anomalies	P	33	2	3	5	5	8	8	2	-	-	-
		M	21	1	1	3	3	4	8	1	-	-	-
		F	12	1	2	2	2	4	-	1	-	-	-
758	Chromosomal anomalies	P	21	5	5	-	5	4	2	-	-	-	-
		M	8	2	1	-	4	1	-	-	-	-	-
		F	13	3	4	-	1	3	2	-	-	-	-
740-759 rem	Other and unspecified congenital anomalies	P	61	8	9	9	8	13	6	2	-	-	6
		M	36	4	8	3	3	8	4	1	-	-	5
		F	25	4	1	6	5	5	2	1	-	-	1
764,765	Prematurity	P	181	42	33	20	23	29	18	9	-	-	7
		M	103	27	18	8	14	21	6	6	-	-	3
		F	78	15	15	12	9	8	12	3	-	-	4
764	Slow fetal growth and fetal malnutrition	P	147	24	27	18	20	26	18	9	-	-	5
		M	77	13	13	6	12	18	6	6	-	-	3
		F	70	11	14	12	8	8	12	3	-	-	2

Table 21 - *continued*

ICD number	Cause of death		Total	Duration of pregnancy (weeks)									
				28-29	30-31	32-33	34-35	36-37	38-39	40	41-42	43 and over	Not stated
765	Disorders relating to short gestation and unspecified low birthweight	P	34	18	6	2	3	3	-	-	-	-	2
		M	26	14	5	2	2	3	-	-	-	-	-
		F	8	4	1	-	1	-	-	-	-	-	2
7650	Extreme immaturity	P	3	2	1	-	-	-	-	-	-	-	-
		M	3	2	1	-	-	-	-	-	-	-	-
		F	.	-	-	-	-	-	-	-	-	-	-
7651	Other preterm infants	P	31	16	5	2	3	3	-	-	-	-	2
		M	23	12	4	2	2	3	-	-	-	-	-
		F	8	4	1	-	1	-	-	-	-	-	2
767	Birth trauma	P	12	-	-	1	1	-	2	4	1	1	2
		F	7	-	-	1	-	-	1	4	-	1	-
7670	Subdural and cerebral haemorrhage	P	12	-	-	1	1	-	2	4	1	1	2
		M	5	-	-	-	1	-	1	-	1	-	2
		F	7	-	-	1	-	-	1	4	-	1	-
768	Intrauterine hypoxia and birth asphyxia	P	1,135	84	91	136	146	181	198	143	86	6	64
		M	612	46	48	71	89	112	94	70	42	5	35
		F	523	38	43	65	57	69	104	73	44	1	29
7680	Death from asphyxia or anoxia before onset of labour or at unspecified time	P	930	71	86	123	134	161	151	88	53	3	60
		M	508	40	44	66	82	101	68	44	27	3	33
		F	422	31	42	57	52	60	83	44	26	-	27
7681	Death from asphyxia or anoxia during labour	P	205	13	5	13	12	20	47	55	33	3	4
		M	104	6	4	5	7	11	26	26	15	2	2
		F	101	7	1	8	5	9	21	29	18	1	2
7689	Unspecified birth asphyxia in liveborn infant	P	.	-	-	-	-	-	-	-	-	-	-
		M	.	-	-	-	-	-	-	-	-	-	-
		F	.	-	-	-	-	-	-	-	-	-	-
512,514, 516,518, 519,769, 770	Non-infectious respiratory disorders	P	10	-	3	-	2	-	-	1	3	1	-
		M	4	-	-	-	2	-	-	-	2	-	-
		F	6	-	3	-	-	-	-	1	1	1	-
769	Respiratory distress syndrome	P	.	-	-	-	-	-	-	-	-	-	-
		M	.	-	-	-	-	-	-	-	-	-	-
		F	.	-	-	-	-	-	-	-	-	-	-
770	Other respiratory conditions of fetus and newborn	P	10	-	3	-	2	-	-	1	3	1	-
		M	4	-	-	-	2	-	-	-	2	-	-
		F	6	-	3	-	-	-	-	1	1	1	-
001-139, 320-326, 460-511, 513,771	Infections and infectious diseases	P	10	3	3	-	2	-	1	-	-	1	-
		M	7	2	2	-	1	-	1	-	-	1	-
		F	3	1	1	-	1	-	-	-	-	-	-
320-322	Meningitis	P	.	-	-	-	-	-	-	-	-	-	-
		M	.	-	-	-	-	-	-	-	-	-	-
		F	.	-	-	-	-	-	-	-	-	-	-
480-486	Pneumonia	P	.	-	-	-	-	-	-	-	-	-	-
		M	.	-	-	-	-	-	-	-	-	-	-
		F	.	-	-	-	-	-	-	-	-	-	-
771	Infections specific to the perinatal period	P	10	3	3	-	2	-	1	-	-	1	-
		M	7	2	2	-	1	-	1	-	-	1	-
		F	3	1	1	-	1	-	-	-	-	-	-
766, 772-779	Other perinatal causes	P	441	56	61	67	57	62	63	30	24	1	20
		M	225	31	32	29	26	36	37	17	10	1	6
		F	216	25	29	38	31	26	26	13	14	-	14
766	Disorders relating to long gestation and high birthweight	P	9	-	-	-	-	-	-	1	7	1	-
		M	5	-	-	-	-	-	-	1	3	1	-
		F	4	-	-	-	-	-	-	-	4	-	-

Table 21 - *continued*

ICD number	Cause of death		Total	Duration of pregnancy (weeks)									
				28-29	30-31	32-33	34-35	36-37	38-39	40	41-42	43 and over	Not stated
772	Fetal and neonatal	P	14	2	1	2	2	1	3	1	2	-	-
	haemorrhage	M	9	-	1	1	2	1	1	1	2	-	-
		F	5	2	-	1	-	-	2	-	-	-	-
773	Haemolytic disease of	P	16	3	3	3	5	1	1	-	-	-	-
	fetus or newborn, due	M	8	1	1	1	3	1	1	-	-	-	-
	to isoimmunization	F	8	2	2	2	2	-	-	-	-	-	-
7730	Due to Rh	P	10	2	2	2	2	1	1	-	-	-	-
	isoimmunization	M	6	1	1	1	1	1	1	-	-	-	-
		F	4	1	1	1	1	-	-	-	-	-	-
774	Other perinatal jaundice	P	.	-	-	-	-	-	-	-	-	-	-
		M	.	-	-	-	-	-	-	-	-	-	-
		F	.	-	-	-	-	-	-	-	-	-	-
775	Endocrine and metabolic	P	6	-	-	-	-	5	-	1	-	-	-
	disturbances specific	M	2	-	-	-	-	2	-	-	-	-	-
	to the fetus and newborn	F	4	-	-	-	-	3	-	1	-	-	-
7750	Syndrome of 'infant	P	6	-	-	-	-	5	-	1	-	-	-
	to a diabetic mother'	M	2	-	-	-	-	2	-	-	-	-	-
		F	4	-	-	-	-	3	-	1	-	-	-
776	Haematological disorders	P	2	-	-	-	-	1	1	-	-	-	-
	of fetus and newborn	M	1	-	-	-	-	-	1	-	-	-	-
		F	1	-	-	-	-	1	-	-	-	-	-
777	Perinatal disorders of	P	.	-	-	-	-	-	-	-	-	-	-
	digestive system	M	.	-	-	-	-	-	-	-	-	-	-
		F	.	-	-	-	-	-	-	-	-	-	-
778	Conditions involving the	P	20	5	6	5	1	2	1	-	-	-	-
	integument and	M	10	3	3	1	1	1	1	-	-	-	-
	temperature regulation	F	10	2	3	4	-	1	-	-	-	-	-
	of fetus and newborn												
779	Other and ill-defined	P	374	46	51	57	49	52	57	27	15	-	20
	conditions originating	M	190	27	27	26	20	31	33	15	5	-	6
	in the perinatal period	F	184	19	24	31	29	21	24	12	10	-	14
7799	Unspecified perinatal	P	363	45	51	53	49	50	57	24	14	-	20
	conditions	M	184	26	27	24	20	30	33	13	5	-	6
		F	179	19	24	29	29	20	24	11	9	-	14
4275, 428, 584-586, 780-799, 800-999	Ill-defined conditions, modes of death, injury and poisoning	P	2	-	-	-	-	-	-	1	1	-	-
		M	2	-	-	-	-	-	-	1	1	-	-
		F	.	-	-	-	-	-	-	-	-	-	-
798	Sudden death, cause	P	.	-	-	-	-	-	-	-	-	-	-
	unknown	M	.	-	-	-	-	-	-	-	-	-	-
		F	.	-	-	-	-	-	-	-	-	-	-
7980	Sudden infant death	P	.	-	-	-	-	-	-	-	-	-	-
	syndrome	M	.	-	-	-	-	-	-	-	-	-	-
		F	.	-	-	-	-	-	-	-	-	-	-
760-763	Maternal conditions	P	627	72	75	71	81	97	97	61	37	1	35
	certified as fetal	M	345	39	43	45	50	48	52	34	16	-	18
		F	282	33	32	26	31	49	45	27	21	1	17
001-E999 rem	Other fetal causes	P	14	1	6	3	1	-	1	1	-	-	1
		M	8	1	4	2	1	-	-	-	-	-	-
		F	6	-	2	1	-	-	1	1	-	-	1
7996	No fetal cause	P	1,111	124	134	133	135	184	193	100	59	3	46
		M	602	63	83	74	75	104	96	57	29	-	21
		F	509	61	51	59	60	80	97	43	30	3	25
	Maternal mentions	P	1,342	173	171	193	187	220	193	92	54	5	54
		M	762	89	102	98	108	141	104	60	27	4	29
		F	580	84	69	95	79	79	89	32	27	1	25

Table 21 - *continued*

ICD number	Cause of death		Total	28-29	30-31	32-33	34-35	36-37	38-39	40	41-42	43 and over	Not stated
642, 7600	Hypertension	P	254	49	42	34	39	29	27	18	8	-	8
		M	136	23	21	16	22	18	13	13	6	-	4
		F	118	26	21	18	17	11	14	5	2	-	4
647,648, 760 rem	Other maternal conditions which may be unrelated to the present pregnancy	P	30	2	2	3	2	9	6	2	-	1	3
		M	11	-	-	1	-	5	3	-	-	1	1
		F	19	2	2	2	2	4	3	2	-	-	2
761	Maternal complications in pregnancy	P	.	-	-	-	-	-	-	-	-	-	-
		M	.	-	-	-	-	-	-	-	-	-	-
		F	.	-	-	-	-	-	-	-	-	-	-
762	Complications of placenta, cord and membranes	P	.	-	-	-	-	-	-	-	-	-	-
		M	.	-	-	-	-	-	-	-	-	-	-
		F	.	-	-	-	-	-	-	-	-	-	-
651, 7615	Multiple pregnancy	P	44	8	1	5	9	9	8	1	-	-	3
		M	26	4	1	4	6	4	3	1	-	-	3
		F	18	4	-	1	3	5	5	-	-	-	-
630-639, 643,646, 650,663, 655-658, 670-676, 761-762 rem	Other maternal complications of pregnancy, placenta, cord or membranes	P	333	39	34	36	41	50	62	36	23	1	11
		M	180	22	21	18	17	36	32	19	10	1	4
		F	153	17	13	18	24	14	30	17	13	-	7
7622	Other and unspecified morphological and functional abnormalities of placenta	P	.	-	-	-	-	-	-	-	-	-	-
		M	.	-	-	-	-	-	-	-	-	-	-
		F	.	-	-	-	-	-	-	-	-	-	-
7624	Prolapsed cord	P	.	-	-	-	-	-	-	-	-	-	-
		M	.	-	-	-	-	-	-	-	-	-	-
		F	.	-	-	-	-	-	-	-	-	-	-
7625	Other compression of umbilical cord	P	.	-	-	-	-	-	-	-	-	-	-
		M	.	-	-	-	-	-	-	-	-	-	-
		F	.	-	-	-	-	-	-	-	-	-	-
640,641, 7620, 7621	Maternal antepartum haemorrhage	P	506	62	69	95	77	87	60	24	13	-	19
		M	303	31	40	52	50	54	36	21	6	-	13
		F	203	31	29	43	27	33	24	3	7	-	6
7620	Placenta praevia	P	.	-	-	-	-	-	-	-	-	-	-
		M	.	-	-	-	-	-	-	-	-	-	-
		F	.	-	-	-	-	-	-	-	-	-	-
7621	Other forms of placental separation and haemorrhage	P	.	-	-	-	-	-	-	-	-	-	-
		M	.	-	-	-	-	-	-	-	-	-	-
		F	.	-	-	-	-	-	-	-	-	-	-
644,645, 652-654, 659-662, 664-669, 7610, 7617,763	Complications of presentation, labour and delivery	P	45	-	4	5	5	6	8	4	7	3	3
		M	23	-	4	3	1	3	3	2	4	2	1
		F	22	-	-	2	4	3	5	2	3	1	2
763	Other complications of labour and delivery	P	.	-	-	-	-	-	-	-	-	-	-
		M	.	-	-	-	-	-	-	-	-	-	-
		F	.	-	-	-	-	-	-	-	-	-	-
001- E999 rem	Other maternal conditions	P	130	13	19	15	14	30	22	7	3	-	7
		M	83	9	15	4	12	21	14	4	1	-	3
		F	47	4	4	11	2	9	8	3	2	-	4
7996	No maternal cause	P	2,308	241	251	269	276	353	392	248	151	10	117
		M	1,206	133	140	143	153	193	188	125	71	3	57
		F	1,102	108	111	126	123	160	204	123	80	7	60

England and Wales

Table 22 Stillbirths, infant deaths and live births: numbers and rates per 1,000 total/live births: birthweight by age of mother, 1986

Age of mother	Birthweight (grams)	Stillbirths		Early neonatal deaths		Late neonatal deaths		Postneonatal deaths		Infant deaths		Live births
		Number	Rate	Number	Rate	Number	Rate	Number	Rate	Number	Rate	Number
All ages	**All weights**	**3,549**	**5.3**	**2,789**	**4.2**	**660**	**1.0**	**2,760**	**4.2**	**6,209**	**9.4**	**661,018**
	Under 2,500	2,208	46.1	1,933	42.3	349	7.6	706	15.4	2,988	65.3	45,728
	Under 1,500	1,118	155.3	1,369	225.1	226	37.2	244	40.1	1,839	302.4	6,081
	1,500-1,999	501	53.3	298	33.5	59	6.6	186	20.9	543	61.1	8,894
	2,000-2,499	589	18.8	266	8.6	64	2.1	276	9.0	606	19.7	30,753
	2,500-2,999	529	4.4	269	2.2	96	0.8	591	4.9	956	8.0	119,810
	3,000-3,499	466	1.8	282	1.1	121	0.5	816	3.2	1,219	4.8	252,035
	3,500 and over	318	1.3	211	0.9	86	0.4	636	2.6	933	3.8	242,821
	Not stated	28	42.9	94	150.6	8	12.8	11	17.6	113	181.1	624
Under 20	**All weights**	**367**	**6.4**	**361**	**6.3**	**74**	**1.3**	**412**	**7.2**	**847**	**14.8**	**57,406**
	Under 2,500	246	44.1	271	50.8	45	8.4	103	19.3	419	78.5	5,336
	Under 1,500	131	148.7	207	276.0	26	34.7	29	38.7	262	349.3	750
	1,500-1,999	59	50.7	40	36.2	8	7.2	34	30.8	82	74.3	1,104
	2,000-2,499	56	15.8	24	6.9	11	3.2	40	11.5	75	21.5	3,482
	2,500-2,999	46	3.7	35	2.8	14	1.1	112	9.0	161	12.9	12,434
	3,000-3,499	49	2.2	26	1.2	11	0.5	122	5.4	159	7.1	22,505
	3,500 and over	24	1.4	16	0.9	3	0.2	73	4.3	92	5.4	17,071
	Not stated	2	32.3	13	216.7	1	16.7	2	33.3	16	266.7	60
20-24	**All weights**	**1,017**	**5.3**	**806**	**4.2**	**203**	**1.1**	**959**	**5.0**	**1,968**	**10.2**	**192,064**
	Under 2,500	675	46.8	581	42.3	96	7.0	226	16.4	903	65.7	13,745
	Under 1,500	351	165.6	409	231.2	62	35.0	76	43.0	547	309.2	1,769
	1,500-1,999	146	53.1	87	33.4	16	6.1	64	24.6	167	64.2	2,602
	2,000-2,499	178	18.6	85	9.1	18	1.9	86	9.2	189	20.2	9,374
	2,500-2,999	146	3.9	60	1.6	33	0.9	197	5.2	290	7.7	37,576
	3,000-3,499	116	1.5	83	1.1	43	0.6	303	4.0	429	5.7	75,174
	3,500 and over	74	1.1	52	0.8	29	0.4	228	3.5	309	4.7	65,389
	Not stated	6	32.3	30	166.7	2	11.1	5	27.8	37	205.6	180
25-29	**All weights**	**1,098**	**4.8**	**850**	**3.7**	**224**	**1.0**	**814**	**3.6**	**1,888**	**8.2**	**229,035**
	Under 2,500	666	44.7	576	40.5	113	7.9	221	15.5	910	64.0	14,225
	Under 1,500	327	151.6	407	222.4	75	41.0	84	45.9	566	309.3	1,830
	1,500-1,999	147	50.6	89	32.2	22	8.0	54	19.6	165	59.8	2,761
	2,000-2,499	192	19.5	80	8.3	16	1.7	83	8.6	179	18.6	9,634
	2,500-2,999	164	4.1	95	2.4	29	0.7	168	4.3	292	7.4	39,429
	3,000-3,499	160	1.8	87	1.0	41	0.5	241	2.7	369	4.2	87,840
	3,500 and over	101	1.2	74	0.8	36	0.4	182	2.1	292	3.3	87,351
	Not stated	7	35.5	18	94.7	5	26.3	2	10.5	25	131.6	190
30-34	**All weights**	**680**	**5.2**	**492**	**3.8**	**105**	**0.8**	**387**	**3.0**	**984**	**7.6**	**129,487**
	Under 2,500	392	44.5	322	38.2	61	7.2	102	12.1	485	57.6	8,420
	Under 1,500	195	148.7	220	197.1	42	37.6	40	35.8	302	270.6	1,116
	1,500-1,999	101	58.2	53	32.4	8	4.9	17	10.4	78	47.7	1,634
	2,000-2,499	96	16.6	49	8.6	11	1.9	45	7.9	105	18.5	5,670
	2,500-2,999	113	5.2	50	2.3	14	0.7	79	3.7	143	6.7	21,411
	3,000-3,499	96	2.0	54	1.1	20	0.4	97	2.0	171	3.6	47,810
	3,500 and over	76	1.5	46	0.9	10	0.2	108	2.1	164	3.2	51,720
	Not stated	3	23.3	20	158.7	-	-	1	7.9	21	166.7	126
35 and over	**All weights**	**387**	**7.2**	**280**	**5.3**	**54**	**1.0**	**188**	**3.5**	**522**	**9.8**	**53,025**
	Under 2,500	229	54.1	183	45.7	34	8.5	54	13.5	271	67.7	4,002
	Under 1,500	114	156.2	126	204.5	21	34.1	15	24.4	162	263.0	616
	1,500-1,999	48	57.1	29	36.6	5	6.3	17	21.4	51	64.3	793
	2,000-2,499	67	25.2	28	10.8	8	3.1	22	8.5	58	22.4	2,593
	2,500-2,999	60	6.7	29	3.2	6	0.7	35	3.9	70	7.8	8,960
	3,000-3,499	45	2.4	32	1.7	6	0.3	53	2.8	91	4.9	18,705
	3,500 and over	43	2.0	23	1.1	8	0.4	45	2.1	76	3.6	21,290
	Not stated	10	128.2	13	191.2	-	-	1	14.7	14	205.9	68

Table 23 Stillbirths, infant deaths and live births - numbers and rates per 1,000 total/live births : birthweight by parity (legitimate only), 1986 — **England and Wales**

Parity	Birthweight (grams)	Stillbirths		Early neonatal deaths		Late neonatal deaths		Postneonatal deaths		Infant deaths		Live births
		Number	Rate	Number	Rate	Number	Rate	Number	Rate	Number	Rate	Number
All	All weights	3,549	5.3	2,789	4.2	660	1.0	2,760	4.2	6,209	9.4	661,018
	Under 2,500	2,208	46.1	1,933	42.3	349	7.6	706	15.4	2,988	65.3	45,728
	Under 1,500	1,118	155.3	1,369	225.1	226	37.2	244	40.1	1,839	302.4	6,081
	1,500-1,999	501	53.3	298	33.5	59	6.6	186	20.9	543	61.1	8,894
	2,000-2,499	589	18.8	266	8.6	64	2.1	276	9.0	606	19.7	30,753
	2,500-2,999	529	4.4	269	2.2	96	0.8	591	4.9	956	8.0	119,810
	3,000-3,499	466	1.8	282	1.1	121	0.5	816	3.2	1,219	4.8	252,035
	3,500 and over	318	1.3	211	0.9	86	0.4	636	2.6	933	3.8	242,821
	Not stated	28	42.9	94	150.6	8	12.8	11	17.6	113	181.1	624
All legitimate	All weights	2,600	5.0	1,991	3.8	470	0.9	1,901	3.7	4,362	8.4	519,673
	Under 2,500	1,562	45.2	1,328	40.3	249	7.6	465	14.1	2,042	62.0	32,961
	Under 1,500	787	159.3	912	219.6	152	36.6	151	36.4	1,215	292.6	4,153
	1,500-1,999	347	51.5	220	34.4	47	7.4	116	18.2	383	60.0	6,387
	2,000-2,499	428	18.7	196	8.7	50	2.2	198	8.8	444	19.8	22,421
	2,500-2,999	398	4.4	206	2.3	68	0.8	392	4.4	666	7.4	89,747
	3,000-3,499	361	1.8	218	1.1	84	0.4	561	2.8	863	4.4	197,124
	3,500 and over	262	1.3	171	0.9	63	0.3	475	2.4	709	3.6	199,381
	Not stated	17	35.6	68	147.8	6	13.0	8	17.4	82	178.3	460
0	All weights	1,141	5.5	830	4.0	195	0.9	538	2.6	1,563	7.6	205,586
	Under 2,500	721	43.5	569	35.9	120	7.6	167	10.5	856	54.0	15,845
	Under 1,500	385	155.6	425	203.4	78	37.3	69	33.0	572	273.8	2,089
	1,500-1,999	158	47.9	68	21.6	19	6.0	36	11.5	123	39.1	3,143
	2,000-2,499	178	16.5	76	7.2	23	2.2	62	5.8	161	15.2	10,613
	2,500-2,999	167	4.1	80	2.0	30	0.7	100	2.5	210	5.2	40,361
	3,000-3,499	154	1.9	99	1.2	28	0.3	164	2.0	291	3.6	81,387
	3,500 and over	94	1.4	61	0.9	14	0.2	102	1.5	177	2.6	67,835
	Not stated	5	30.7	21	132.9	3	19.0	5	31.6	29	183.5	158
1	All weights	731	3.9	648	3.4	159	0.8	725	3.8	1,532	8.1	188,539
	Under 2,500	436	43.6	413	43.2	82	8.6	175	18.3	670	70.1	9,560
	Under 1,500	203	152.1	259	228.8	53	46.8	48	42.4	360	318.0	1,132
	1,500-1,999	108	57.1	84	47.1	17	9.5	50	28.0	151	84.6	1,785
	2,000-2,499	125	18.5	70	10.5	12	1.8	77	11.6	159	23.9	6,643
	2,500-2,999	105	3.6	73	2.5	17	0.6	166	5.7	256	8.8	29,038
	3,000-3,499	103	1.5	75	1.1	35	0.5	210	3.0	320	4.5	70,562
	3,500 and over	80	1.0	67	0.8	24	0.3	173	2.2	264	3.3	79,219
	Not stated	7	41.9	20	125.0	1	6.2	1	6.2	22	137.5	160
2	All weights	403	4.9	294	3.6	71	0.9	405	5.0	770	9.5	81,460
	Under 2,500	232	48.7	200	44.1	27	6.0	74	16.3	301	66.4	4,532
	Under 1,500	117	180.6	126	237.3	15	28.2	21	39.5	162	305.1	531
	1,500-1,999	49	52.4	41	46.3	7	7.9	20	22.6	68	76.7	886
	2,000-2,499	66	20.7	33	10.6	5	1.6	33	10.6	71	22.8	3,115
	2,500-2,999	65	5.1	27	2.1	12	1.0	81	6.4	120	9.5	12,588
	3,000-3,499	61	2.1	22	0.7	16	0.5	109	3.7	147	5.0	29,606
	3,500 and over	44	1.3	26	0.8	15	0.4	141	4.1	182	5.3	34,646
	Not stated	1	11.2	19	215.9	1	11.4	-	-	20	227.3	88
3 and over	All weights	325	7.3	219	5.0	45	1.0	233	5.3	497	11.3	44,088
	Under 2,500	173	54.1	146	48.3	20	6.6	49	16.2	215	71.1	3,024
	Under 1,500	82	169.8	102	254.4	6	15.0	13	32.4	121	301.7	401
	1,500-1,999	32	52.9	27	47.1	4	7.0	10	17.5	41	71.6	573
	2,000-2,499	59	28.0	17	8.3	10	4.9	26	12.7	53	25.9	2,050
	2,500-2,999	61	7.8	26	3.4	9	1.2	45	5.8	80	10.3	7,760
	3,000-3,499	43	2.8	22	1.4	5	0.3	78	5.0	105	6.7	15,569
	3,500 and over	44	2.5	17	1.0	10	0.6	59	3.3	86	4.9	17,681
	Not stated	4	69.0	8	148.1	1	18.5	2	37.0	11	203.7	54
Illegitimate	All weights	949	6.7	798	5.6	190	1.3	859	6.1	1,847	13.1	141,345
	Under 2,500	646	48.2	605	47.4	100	7.8	241	18.9	946	74.1	12,767
	Under 1,500	331	146.5	457	237.0	74	38.4	93	48.2	624	323.7	1,928
	1,500-1,999	154	57.9	78	31.1	12	4.8	70	27.9	160	63.8	2,507
	2,000-2,499	161	19.0	70	8.4	14	1.7	78	9.4	162	19.4	8,332
	2,500-2,999	131	4.3	63	2.1	28	0.9	199	6.6	290	9.6	30,063
	3,000-3,499	105	1.9	64	1.2	37	0.7	255	4.6	356	6.5	54,911
	3,500 and over	56	1.3	40	0.9	23	0.5	161	3.7	224	5.2	43,440
	Not stated	11	62.9	26	158.5	2	12.2	3	18.3	31	189.0	164

Table 24   Stillbirths, infant deaths and live births - numbers and rates per 1,000 total/live births : birthweight by social class (legitimate only), 1986   **England and Wales**

Social class (legiti-mate only)	Birthweight (grams)	Stillbirths		Early neonatal deaths		Late neonatal deaths		Postneonatal deaths		Infant deaths		Live births
		Number	Rate	Number	Rate	Number	Rate	Number	Rate	Number	Rate	Number
All legitimate	All weights	2,600	5.0	1,991	3.8	470	0.9	1,901	3.7	4,362	8.4	519,673
	Under 2,500	1,562	45.2	1,328	40.3	249	7.6	465	14.1	2,042	62.0	32,961
	Under 1,500	787	159.3	912	219.6	152	36.6	151	36.4	1,215	292.6	4,153
	1,500-1,999	347	51.5	220	34.4	47	7.4	116	18.2	383	60.0	6,387
	2,000-2,499	428	18.7	196	8.7	50	2.2	198	8.8	444	19.8	22,421
	2,500-2,999	398	4.4	206	2.3	68	0.8	392	4.4	666	7.4	89,747
	3,000-3,499	361	1.8	218	1.1	84	0.4	561	2.8	863	4.4	197,124
	3,500 and over	262	1.3	171	0.9	63	0.3	475	2.4	709	3.6	199,381
	Not stated	17	35.6	68	147.8	6	13.0	8	17.4	82	178.3	460
I-V	All weights	2,439	4.9	1,847	3.7	442	0.9	1,737	3.5	4,026	8.1	495,880
	Under 2,500	1,454	45.2	1,232	40.1	234	7.6	430	14.0	1,896	61.7	30,740
	Under 1,500	734	161.8	848	223.1	143	37.6	140	36.8	1,131	297.5	3,800
	1,500-1,999	328	52.5	203	34.3	44	7.4	109	18.4	356	60.2	5,920
	2,000-2,499	392	18.3	181	8.6	47	2.2	181	8.6	409	19.5	21,020
	2,500-2,999	386	4.5	192	2.2	64	0.7	359	4.2	615	7.2	85,860
	3,000-3,499	339	1.8	207	1.1	81	0.4	510	2.7	798	4.3	187,250
	3,500 and over	245	1.3	153	0.8	57	0.3	430	2.2	640	3.3	191,700
	Not stated	15	44.7	63	196.4	6	18.7	8	24.9	77	240.1	320
I	All weights	150	3.7	143	3.5	24	0.6	109	2.7	276	6.8	40,810
	Under 2,500	89	38.1	91	40.6	14	6.2	26	11.6	131	58.4	2,240
	Under 1,500	50	122.4	57	158.9	9	25.1	9	25.1	75	209.1	360
	1,500-1,999	22	62.6	16	48.6	2	6.1	4	12.1	22	66.8	330
	2,000-2,499	17	10.8	18	11.6	3	1.9	13	8.4	34	21.9	1,560
	2,500-2,999	25	4.1	14	2.3	3	0.5	23	3.8	40	6.6	6,060
	3,000-3,499	21	1.3	20	1.3	2	0.1	31	2.0	53	3.4	15,550
	3,500 and over	14	0.8	16	0.9	5	0.3	28	1.7	49	2.9	16,950
	Not stated	1	1,000.0	2	..	-	-	1	..	3	..	-
II	All weights	478	4.0	387	3.2	98	0.8	353	3.0	838	7.0	119,300
	Under 2,500	264	41.8	254	42.0	55	9.1	73	12.1	382	63.2	6,050
	Under 1,500	116	132.8	184	243.0	37	48.9	21	27.7	242	319.6	760
	1,500-1,999	68	55.2	41	35.2	5	4.3	15	12.9	61	52.4	1,160
	2,000-2,499	80	19.0	29	7.0	13	3.2	37	9.0	79	19.1	4,130
	2,500-2,999	77	4.1	41	2.2	15	0.8	73	3.9	129	6.9	18,740
	3,000-3,499	84	1.9	49	1.1	13	0.3	110	2.5	172	3.9	44,590
	3,500 and over	49	1.0	27	0.5	14	0.3	95	1.9	136	2.7	49,820
	Not stated	4	38.6	16	160.5	1	10.0	2	20.1	19	190.6	100
IIIN	All weights	267	4.8	198	3.6	39	0.7	168	3.0	405	7.3	55,220
	Under 2,500	171	55.8	121	41.8	22	7.6	48	16.6	191	66.0	2,890
	Under 1,500	81	213.4	75	251.1	13	43.5	20	67.0	108	361.7	300
	1,500-1,999	50	69.9	19	28.6	7	10.5	12	18.1	38	57.2	660
	2,000-2,499	40	20.3	27	14.0	2	1.0	16	8.3	45	23.3	1,930
	2,500-2,999	37	4.3	22	2.6	7	0.8	28	3.3	57	6.6	8,610
	3,000-3,499	32	1.5	21	1.0	4	0.2	49	2.3	74	3.5	21,360
	3,500 and over	25	1.1	30	1.3	5	0.2	41	1.8	76	3.4	22,340
	Not stated	2	91.6	4	201.7	1	50.4	2	100.8	7	352.9	20
IIIM	All weights	939	5.2	672	3.7	169	0.9	616	3.4	1,457	8.1	179,500
	Under 2,500	571	45.0	461	38.0	87	7.2	156	12.9	704	58.1	12,120
	Under 1,500	299	165.8	324	215.3	51	33.9	56	37.2	431	286.4	1,510
	1,500-1,999	116	49.8	77	34.8	20	9.0	46	20.8	143	64.6	2,210
	2,000-2,499	156	18.2	60	7.1	16	1.9	54	6.4	130	15.5	8,400
	2,500-2,999	153	4.7	67	2.1	19	0.6	124	3.8	210	6.5	32,330
	3,000-3,499	117	1.7	66	1.0	37	0.6	186	2.8	289	4.3	67,260
	3,500 and over	91	1.3	54	0.8	25	0.4	148	2.2	227	3.4	67,690
	Not stated	7	64.9	24	238.0	1	9.9	2	19.8	27	267.7	100
IV	All weights	419	5.7	310	4.3	81	1.1	344	4.7	735	10.1	72,890
	Under 2,500	253	46.2	201	38.5	41	7.9	91	17.4	333	63.8	5,220
	Under 1,500	131	164.8	138	207.8	25	37.6	27	40.7	190	286.1	660
	1,500-1,999	49	40.7	32	27.7	7	6.1	21	18.2	60	52.0	1,160
	2,000-2,499	73	21.0	31	9.1	9	2.6	43	12.6	83	24.4	3,400
	2,500-2,999	63	4.4	38	2.7	14	1.0	72	5.1	124	8.8	14,160
	3,000-3,499	59	2.1	38	1.4	17	0.6	94	3.3	149	5.3	28,100
	3,500 and over	43	1.7	21	0.8	7	0.3	86	3.4	114	4.5	25,340
	Not stated	1	14.0	12	169.9	2	28.3	1	14.2	15	212.3	70

Note: Figures by social class for all live births are derived from a 10 per cent sample and have been grossed up to agree with the numbers of legitimate live births by maternal age and parity derived from the 100 per cent processing of birth registrations. Figures may not add to totals due to rounding.

Table 24 - *continued*

Social class (legiti- mate only)	Birthweight (grams)	Stillbirths		Early neonatal deaths		Late neonatal deaths		Postneonatal deaths		Infant deaths		Live births
		Number	Rate	Number	Rate	Number	Rate	Number	Rate	Number	Rate	Number
V	All weights	186	6.6	137	4.9	31	1.1	147	5.2	315	11.2	28,170
	Under 2,500	106	45.6	104	46.8	15	6.8	36	16.2	155	69.8	2,220
	Under 1,500	57	207.1	70	320.8	8	36.7	7	32.1	85	389.5	220
	1,500-1,999	23	55.6	18	46.0	3	7.7	11	28.1	32	81.8	390
	2,000-2,499	26	15.9	16	9.9	4	2.5	18	11.2	38	23.6	1,610
	2,500-2,999	31	5.2	10	1.7	6	1.0	39	6.5	55	9.2	5,960
	3,000-3,499	26	2.5	13	1.3	8	0.8	40	3.8	61	5.9	10,400
	3,500 and over	23	2.4	5	0.5	1	0.1	32	3.3	38	4.0	9,560
	Not stated	-	-	5	168.2	1	33.6	-	-	6	201.8	30
Other	All weights	161	6.7	144	6.1	28	1.2	164	6.9	336	14.1	23,790
	Under 2,500	108	65.0	96	61.8	15	9.7	35	22.5	146	94.0	1,550
	Under 1,500	53	218.8	64	338.2	9	47.6	11	58.1	84	443.9	190
	1,500-1,999	19	61.9	17	59.0	3	10.4	7	24.3	27	93.8	290
	2,000-2,499	36	32.4	15	13.9	3	2.8	17	15.8	35	32.5	1,080
	2,500-2,999	12	2.8	14	3.3	4	0.9	33	7.7	51	11.9	4,280
	3,000-3,499	22	2.5	11	1.2	3	0.3	51	5.8	65	7.4	8,800
	3,500 and over	17	1.9	18	2.0	6	0.7	45	5.0	69	7.6	9,070
	Not stated	2	21.8	5	55.8	-	-	-	-	5	55.8	90

Note: Figures by social class for all live births are derived from a 10 per cent sample and have been grossed up to agree with the numbers of legitimate live births by maternal age and parity derived from the 100 per cent processing of birth registrations. Figures may not add to totals due to rounding.

Table 25 **Stillbirths, infant deaths and live births - numbers and rates per 1,000 total/live births : birthweight by place of confinement, 1986** **England and Wales**

Place of confinement of mother	Birthweight (grams)	Stillbirths		Early neonatal deaths		Late neonatal deaths		Postneonatal deaths		Infant deaths		Live births
		Number	Rate	Number	Rate	Number	Rate	Number	Rate	Number	Rate	Number
Total	All weights	3,549	5.3	2,789	4.2	660	1.0	2,760	4.2	6,209	9.4	661,018
	Under 2,500	2,208	46.1	1,933	42.3	349	7.6	706	15.4	2,988	65.3	45,728
	Under 1,500	1,118	155.3	1,369	225.1	226	37.2	244	40.1	1,839	302.4	6,081
	1,500-1,999	501	53.3	298	33.5	59	6.6	186	20.9	543	61.1	8,894
	2,000-2,499	589	18.8	266	8.6	64	2.1	276	9.0	606	19.7	30,753
	2,500-2,999	529	4.4	269	2.2	96	0.8	591	4.9	956	8.0	119,810
	3,000-3,499	466	1.8	282	1.1	121	0.5	816	3.2	1,219	4.8	252,035
	3,500 and over	318	1.3	211	0.9	86	0.4	636	2.6	933	3.8	242,821
	Not stated	28	42.9	94	150.6	8	12.8	11	17.6	113	181.1	624
NHS hospital A	All weights	15	1.0	20	1.3	4	0.3	55	3.7	79	5.3	14,892
	Under 2,500	4	15.0	5	19.1	-	-	1	3.8	6	22.9	262
	Under 1,500	1	100.0	2	222.2	-	-	-	-	2	222.2	9
	1,500-1,999	-	-	2	87.0	-	-	-	-	2	87.0	23
	2,000-2,499	3	12.9	1	4.3	-	-	1	4.3	2	8.7	230
	2,500-2,999	4	2.0	5	2.5	1	0.5	10	5.1	16	8.2	1,963
	3,000-3,499	5	0.8	3	0.5	3	0.5	24	3.9	30	4.9	6,098
	3,500 and over	2	0.3	3	0.5	-	-	20	3.1	23	3.5	6,552
	Not stated	-	-	4	235.3	-	-	-	-	4	235.3	17
NHS hospital B	All weights	3,432	5.4	2,698	4.3	639	1.0	2,644	4.2	5,981	9.5	632,309
	Under 2,500	2,130	45.4	1,880	42.0	344	7.7	689	15.4	2,913	65.1	44,741
	Under 1,500	1,077	153.6	1,331	224.3	222	37.4	241	40.6	1,794	302.3	5,935
	1,500-1,999	479	51.9	291	33.3	58	6.6	182	20.8	531	60.7	8,751
	2,000-2,499	574	18.7	258	8.6	64	2.1	266	8.9	588	19.6	30,055
	2,500-2,999	521	4.5	257	2.2	91	0.8	570	4.9	918	7.9	115,741
	3,000-3,499	449	1.9	275	1.1	112	0.5	772	3.2	1,159	4.8	240,861
	3,500 and over	309	1.3	205	0.9	84	0.4	602	2.6	891	3.9	230,484
	Not stated	23	45.5	81	168.0	8	16.6	11	22.8	100	207.5	482
Other hospital	All weights	28	3.8	13	1.8	7	1.0	26	3.6	46	6.3	7,283
	Under 2,500	18	52.6	7	21.6	2	6.2	8	24.7	17	52.5	324
	Under 1,500	6	150.0	4	117.6	2	58.8	1	29.4	7	205.9	34
	1,500-1,999	6	101.7	3	56.6	-	-	2	37.7	5	94.3	53
	2,000-2,499	6	24.7	-	-	-	-	5	21.1	5	21.1	237
	2,500-2,999	1	0.9	3	2.8	1	0.9	4	3.7	8	7.5	1,070
	3,000-3,499	6	2.1	-	-	2	0.7	8	2.9	10	3.6	2,792
	3,500 and over	3	1.0	2	0.7	2	0.7	6	2.0	10	3.3	3,035
	Not stated	-	-	1	16.1	-	-	-	-	1	16.1	62
At home	All weights	58	9.6	46	7.7	9	1.5	31	5.2	86	14.3	6,006
	Under 2,500	46	123.7	31	95.1	3	9.2	7	21.5	41	125.8	326
	Under 1,500	27	252.3	26	325.0	2	25.0	2	25.0	30	375.0	80
	1,500-1,999	15	227.3	1	19.6	1	19.6	2	39.2	4	78.4	51
	2,000-2,499	4	20.1	4	20.5	-	-	3	15.4	7	35.9	195
	2,500-2,999	2	2.2	3	3.3	2	2.2	7	7.7	12	13.2	908
	3,000-3,499	6	2.8	4	1.9	4	1.9	10	4.8	18	8.6	2,103
	3,500 and over	3	1.1	1	0.4	-	-	7	2.7	8	3.1	2,613
	Not stated	1	17.5	7	125.0	-	-	-	-	7	125.0	56
Elsewhere	All weights	16	29.4	12	22.7	1	1.9	4	7.6	17	32.2	528
	Under 2,500	10	117.6	10	133.3	-	-	1	13.3	11	146.7	75
	Under 1,500	7	233.3	6	260.9	-	-	-	-	6	260.9	23
	1,500-1,999	1	58.8	1	62.5	-	-	-	-	1	62.5	16
	2,000-2,499	2	52.6	3	83.3	-	-	1	27.8	4	111.1	36
	2,500-2,999	1	7.8	1	7.8	1	7.8	-	-	2	15.6	128
	3,000-3,499	-	-	-	-	-	-	2	11.0	2	11.0	181
	3,500 and over	1	7.2	-	-	-	-	1	7.3	1	7.3	137
	Not stated	4	363.6	1	142.9	-	-	-	-	1	142.9	7

Table 26 **Stillbirths, infant deaths and live births - numbers and rates per 1,000 total/live births : birthweight by country of birth of mother, 1986** **England and Wales**

Country of birth of mother	Birthweight (grams)	Stillbirths		Early neonatal deaths		Late neonatal deaths		Postneonatal deaths		Infant deaths		Live births
		Number	Rate	Number	Rate	Number	Rate	Number	Rate	Number	Rate	Number
All	All weights	3,549	5.3	2,789	4.2	660	1.0	2,760	4.2	6,209	9.4	661,018
	Under 2,500	2,208	46.1	1,933	42.3	349	7.6	706	15.4	2,988	65.3	45,728
	Under 1,500	1,118	155.3	1,369	225.1	226	37.2	244	40.1	1,839	302.4	6,081
	1,500-1,999	501	53.3	298	33.5	59	6.6	186	20.9	543	61.1	8,894
	2,000-2,499	589	18.8	266	8.6	64	2.1	276	9.0	606	19.7	30,753
	2,500-2,999	529	4.4	269	2.2	96	0.8	591	4.9	956	8.0	119,810
	3,000-3,499	466	1.8	282	1.1	121	0.5	816	3.2	1,219	4.8	252,035
	3,500 and over	318	1.3	211	0.9	86	0.4	636	2.6	933	3.8	242,821
	Not stated	28	42.9	94	150.6	8	12.8	11	17.6	113	181.1	624
United Kingdom	All weights	3,036	5.2	2,433	4.2	559	1.0	2,438	4.2	5,430	9.4	579,322
	Under 2,500	1,888	46.5	1,702	43.9	292	7.5	612	15.8	2,606	67.3	38,748
	Under 1,500	956	154.4	1,218	232.7	191	36.5	206	39.4	1,615	308.6	5,234
	1,500-1,999	430	53.2	251	32.8	53	6.9	162	21.2	466	60.9	7,650
	2,000-2,499	502	19.0	233	9.0	48	1.9	244	9.4	525	20.3	25,864
	2,500-2,999	447	4.4	221	2.2	75	0.7	508	5.0	804	8.0	100,880
	3,000-3,499	402	1.8	240	1.1	102	0.5	726	3.3	1,068	4.8	220,318
	3,500 and over	275	1.3	186	0.8	83	0.4	584	2.7	853	3.9	218,908
	Not stated	24	48.8	84	179.5	7	15.0	8	17.1	99	211.5	468
Irish Republic	All weights	28	4.5	23	3.7	3	0.5	25	4.0	51	8.2	6,188
	Under 2,500	17	39.4	17	41.0	2	4.8	5	12.0	24	57.8	415
	Under 1,500	3	47.6	12	200.0	1	16.7	1	16.7	14	233.3	60
	1,500-1,999	6	69.8	4	50.0	-	-	2	25.0	6	75.0	80
	2,000-2,499	8	28.3	1	3.6	1	3.6	2	7.3	4	14.5	275
	2,500-2,999	3	3.0	3	3.0	-	-	6	6.1	9	9.1	987
	3,000-3,499	6	2.6	2	0.9	-	-	11	4.9	13	5.7	2,264
	3,500 and over	2	0.8	1	0.4	-	-	3	1.2	4	1.6	2,507
	Not stated	-	-	-	-	1	66.7	-	-	1	66.7	15
Australia, Canada, and New Zealand	All weights	10	4.0	9	3.6	1	0.4	11	4.5	21	8.5	2,470
	Under 2,500	7	48.3	7	50.7	-	-	2	14.5	9	65.2	138
	Under 1,500	3	166.7	4	266.7	-	-	2	133.3	6	400.0	15
	1,500-1,999	2	69.0	2	74.1	-	-	-	-	2	74.1	27
	2,000-2,499	2	20.4	1	10.4	-	-	-	-	1	10.4	96
	2,500-2,999	1	2.7	-	-	1	2.7	3	8.2	4	11.0	364
	3,000-3,499	1	1.1	2	2.1	-	-	3	3.2	5	5.3	944
	3,500 and over	1	1.0	-	-	-	-	3	2.9	3	2.9	1,023
	Not stated	-	-	-	-	-	-	-	-	-	-	1
New Commonwealth and Pakistan	All weights	373	7.0	251	4.8	79	1.5	221	4.2	551	10.5	52,705
	Under 2,500	231	42.3	164	31.4	46	8.8	71	13.6	281	53.8	5,225
	Under 1,500	127	169.1	111	177.9	26	41.7	27	43.3	164	262.8	624
	1,500-1,999	41	43.7	29	32.3	6	6.7	18	20.1	53	59.1	897
	2,000-2,499	63	16.7	24	6.5	14	3.8	26	7.0	64	17.3	3,704
	2,500-2,999	64	4.5	37	2.6	16	1.1	59	4.2	112	8.0	14,078
	3,000-3,499	46	2.2	26	1.3	14	0.7	57	2.7	97	4.7	20,747
	3,500 and over	31	2.5	17	1.3	3	0.2	32	2.5	52	4.1	12,598
	Not stated	1	17.2	7	122.8	-	-	2	35.1	9	157.9	57
Bangladesh	All weights	31	6.5	15	3.2	8	1.7	11	2.3	34	7.2	4,717
	Under 2,500	16	31.4	8	16.2	4	8.1	5	10.1	17	34.4	494
	Under 1,500	6	157.9	5	156.2	2	62.5	2	62.5	9	281.2	32
	1,500-1,999	5	65.8	2	28.2	1	14.1	1	14.1	4	56.3	71
	2,000-2,499	5	12.6	1	2.6	1	2.6	2	5.1	4	10.2	391
	2,500-2,999	3	2.0	1	0.7	3	2.0	4	2.6	8	5.2	1,527
	3,000-3,499	4	2.2	4	2.2	-	-	1	0.6	5	2.8	1,806
	3,500 and over	7	7.9	1	1.1	1	1.1	1	1.1	3	3.4	874
	Not stated	1	58.8	1	62.5	-	-	-	-	1	62.5	16
India	All weights	67	6.3	46	4.3	8	0.8	42	3.9	96	9.0	10,650
	Under 2,500	43	34.4	31	25.7	5	4.1	14	11.6	50	41.4	1,208
	Under 1,500	25	189.4	20	186.9	3	28.0	4	37.4	27	252.3	107
	1,500-1,999	8	39.6	5	25.8	-	-	3	15.5	8	41.2	194
	2,000-2,499	10	10.9	6	6.6	2	2.2	7	7.7	15	16.5	907
	2,500-2,999	13	3.9	9	2.7	1	0.3	13	4.0	23	7.0	3,286
	3,000-3,499	8	1.9	3	0.7	2	0.5	10	2.4	15	3.6	4,203
	3,500 and over	3	1.5	2	1.0	-	-	5	2.6	7	3.6	1,944
	Not stated	-	-	1	111.1	-	-	-	-	1	111.1	9

Table 26 - *continued*

Country of birth of mother	Birthweight (grams)	Stillbirths		Early neonatal deaths		Late neonatal deaths		Postneonatal deaths		Infant deaths		Live births
		Number	Rate	Number	Rate	Number	Rate	Number	Rate	Number	Rate	Number
East African Commonwealth	All weights	49	6.8	35	4.9	16	2.2	21	2.9	72	10.1	7,142
	Under 2,500	35	37.7	23	25.8	11	12.3	7	7.8	41	45.9	893
	Under 1,500	21	185.8	14	152.2	7	76.1	1	10.9	22	239.1	92
	1,500-1,999	7	41.2	7	42.9	1	6.1	4	24.5	12	73.6	163
	2,000-2,499	7	10.9	2	3.1	3	4.7	2	3.1	7	11.0	638
	2,500-2,999	7	3.0	7	3.0	3	1.3	7	3.0	17	7.2	2,353
	3,000-3,499	2	0.8	2	0.8	2	0.8	6	2.3	10	3.8	2,636
	3,500 and over	5	4.0	3	2.4	-	-	1	0.8	4	3.2	1,255
	Not stated	-	-	-	-	-	-	-	-	-	-	5
Rest of Africa	All weights	25	6.7	15	4.1	5	1.4	18	4.9	38	10.3	3,700
	Under 2,500	17	50.6	10	31.3	2	6.3	6	18.8	18	56.4	319
	Under 1,500	7	88.6	10	138.9	1	13.9	6	83.3	17	236.1	72
	1,500-1,999	3	46.2	-	-	1	16.1	-	-	1	16.1	62
	2,000-2,499	7	36.5	-	-	-	-	-	-	-	-	185
	2,500-2,999	4	6.0	2	3.0	2	3.0	2	3.0	6	9.1	662
	3,000-3,499	2	1.4	1	0.7	1	0.7	4	2.8	6	4.1	1,446
	3,500 and over	2	1.6	2	1.6	-	-	5	3.9	7	5.5	1,266
	Not stated	-	-	-	-	-	-	1	142.9	1	142.9	7
Caribbean Commonwealth	All weights	41	8.7	18	3.9	10	2.1	20	4.3	48	10.3	4,674
	Under 2,500	25	55.9	12	28.4	5	11.8	5	11.8	22	52.1	422
	Under 1,500	14	144.3	8	96.4	5	60.2	3	36.1	16	192.8	83
	1,500-1,999	7	77.8	2	24.1	-	-	1	12.0	3	36.1	83
	2,000-2,499	4	15.4	2	7.8	-	-	1	3.9	3	11.7	256
	2,500-2,999	5	4.9	2	2.0	1	1.0	6	6.0	9	8.9	1,006
	3,000-3,499	7	3.7	1	0.5	4	2.1	6	3.2	11	5.8	1,881
	3,500 and over	4	2.9	2	1.5	-	-	3	2.2	5	3.7	1,361
	Not stated	-	-	1	250.0	-	-	-	-	1	250.0	4
Mediterranean Commonwealth	All weights	11	3.9	14	5.0	4	1.4	9	3.2	27	9.7	2,795
	Under 2,500	8	38.5	10	50.0	1	5.0	2	10.0	13	65.0	200
	Under 1,500	4	90.9	10	250.0	-	-	1	25.0	11	275.0	40
	1,500-1,999	2	51.3	-	-	1	27.0	-	-	1	27.0	37
	2,000-2,499	2	16.0	-	-	-	-	1	8.1	1	8.1	123
	2,500-2,999	2	3.6	2	3.6	2	3.6	4	7.2	8	14.4	556
	3,000-3,499	1	0.9	1	0.9	-	-	1	0.9	2	1.9	1,077
	3,500 and over	-	-	-	-	1	1.0	2	2.1	3	3.1	960
	Not stated	-	-	1	500.0	-	-	-	-	1	500.0	2
Remainder of New Commonwealth	All weights	12	2.2	14	2.6	5	0.9	17	3.1	36	6.6	5,468
	Under 2,500	5	12.5	7	17.7	3	7.6	3	7.6	13	32.9	395
	Under 1,500	2	54.1	4	114.3	2	57.1	1	28.6	7	200.0	35
	1,500-1,999	-	-	1	14.9	-	-	-	-	1	14.9	67
	2,000-2,499	3	10.1	2	6.8	1	3.4	2	6.8	5	17.1	293
	2,500-2,999	6	4.8	2	1.6	-	-	2	1.6	4	3.2	1,251
	3,000-3,499	1	0.4	3	1.3	2	0.9	6	2.7	11	4.9	2,249
	3,500 and over	-	-	2	1.3	-	-	6	3.8	8	5.1	1,568
	Not stated	-	-	-	-	-	-	-	-	-	-	5
Pakistan	All weights	137	10.0	94	6.9	23	1.7	83	6.1	200	14.8	13,559
	Under 2,500	82	59.6	63	48.7	15	11.6	29	22.4	107	82.7	1,294
	Under 1,500	48	227.5	40	245.4	6	36.8	9	55.2	55	337.4	163
	1,500-1,999	9	39.3	12	54.5	2	9.1	9	40.9	23	104.5	220
	2,000-2,499	25	26.7	11	12.1	7	7.7	11	12.1	29	31.8	911
	2,500-2,999	24	6.9	12	3.5	4	1.2	21	6.1	37	10.8	3,437
	3,000-3,499	21	3.8	11	2.0	3	0.6	23	4.2	37	6.8	5,449
	3,500 and over	10	3.0	5	1.5	1	0.3	9	2.7	15	4.5	3,370
	Not stated	-	-	3	333.3	-	-	1	111.1	4	444.4	9
Remainder of Europe	All weights	43	4.9	28	3.2	10	1.1	37	4.2	75	8.6	8,749
	Under 2,500	27	50.7	18	35.6	5	9.9	5	9.9	28	55.3	506
	Under 1,500	11	142.9	10	151.5	4	60.6	1	15.2	15	227.3	66
	1,500-1,999	12	101.7	4	37.7	-	-	2	18.9	6	56.6	106
	2,000-2,499	4	11.8	4	12.0	1	3.0	2	6.0	7	21.0	334
	2,500-2,999	7	4.9	3	2.1	2	1.4	12	8.4	17	11.9	1,431
	3,000-3,499	6	1.8	2	0.6	3	0.9	13	3.9	18	5.4	3,312
	3,500 and over	3	0.9	5	1.4	-	-	7	2.0	12	3.4	3,492
	Not stated	-	-	-	-	-	-	-	-	-	-	8

Table 26 - *continued*

Country of birth of mother	Birthweight (grams)	Stillbirths		Early neonatal deaths		Late neonatal deaths		Postneonatal deaths		Infant deaths		Live births
		Number	Rate	Number	Rate	Number	Rate	Number	Rate	Number	Rate	Number
Other	All weights	53	4.6	42	3.7	7	0.6	27	2.4	76	6.6	11,479
	Under 2,500	36	49.9	22	32.1	4	5.8	11	16.0	37	53.9	686
	Under 1,500	17	178.9	11	141.0	4	51.3	7	89.7	22	282.1	78
	1,500-1,999	9	63.8	8	60.6	-	-	2	15.2	10	75.8	132
	2,000-2,499	10	20.6	3	6.3	-	-	2	4.2	5	10.5	476
	2,500-2,999	7	3.4	5	2.4	2	1.0	3	1.5	10	4.9	2,051
	3,000-3,499	4	0.9	10	2.3	1	0.2	5	1.1	16	3.6	4,407
	3,500 and over	6	1.4	2	0.5	-	-	7	1.6	9	2.1	4,260
	Not stated	-	-	3	40.0	-	-	1	13.3	4	53.3	75
Not stated	All weights	6	54.1	3	28.6	1	9.5	1	9.5	5	47.6	105
	Under 2,500	2	166.7	3	300.0	-	-	-	-	3	300.0	10
	Under 1,500	1	200.0	3	750.0	-	-	-	-	3	750.0	4
	1,500-1,999	1	333.3	-	-	-	-	-	-	-	-	2
	2,000-2,499	-	-	-	-	-	-	-	-	-	-	4
	2,500-2,999	-	-	-	-	-	-	-	-	-	-	19
	3,000-3,499	1	22.7	-	-	1	23.3	1	23.3	2	46.5	43
	3,500 and over	-	-	-	-	-	-	-	-	-	-	33
	Not stated	3	1,000.0	-	-	-	-	-	-	-	-	-

Table 27a Stillbirths (a), and neonatal deaths (b) - numbers: **England and Wales**
birthweight by cause of death, 1986

ICD number	Cause of death		Birthweight (grams)										
			All weights	Under 500	500 - 999	1000 - 1499	1500 - 1999	2000 - 2499	2500 - 2999	3000 - 3499	3500 - 3999	4000 and over	Not stated
	All causes Stillbirths	(a)	3,549	72	426	620	501	589	529	466	214	104	28
	Neonatal deaths	(b)	3,449	79	983	533	357	330	365	403	220	77	102
	Fetal mentions	(a)	2,715	59	319	469	406	449	394	359	153	83	24
		(b)	4,368	84	1,157	730	485	451	477	500	263	99	122
740-759	Congenital anomalies	(a)	283	4	50	74	45	41	37	20	7	3	2
		(b)	1,230	5	38	140	186	240	239	216	100	37	29
740	Anencephalus	(a)	41	1	9	14	9	3	2	-	1	1	1
		(b)	26	-	3	6	5	5	4	2	-	-	1
741	Spina bifida	(a)	21	-	2	4	1	6	1	5	2	-	-
		(b)	65	2	-	3	7	13	19	12	7	2	-
7420	Encephalocele	(a)	1	-	-	-	1	-	-	-	-	-	-
		(b)	26	1	-	4	3	6	6	4	1	-	1
742 rem	Other congenital anomalies of central nervous system	(a)	42	-	6	8	4	4	10	8	2	-	-
		(b)	65	-	3	1	15	11	12	12	3	7	1
745	Bulbus cordis anomalies and anomalies of cardiac septal closure	(a)	2	-	1	-	-	1	-	-	-	-	-
		(b)	115	-	1	6	10	18	24	37	12	5	2
746	Other congenital anomalies of heart	(a)	10	-	2	1	2	3	1	-	-	1	-
		(b)	224	1	-	7	10	37	54	64	39	11	1
747	Other congenital anomalies of circulatory system	(a)	1	-	-	-	1	-	-	-	-	-	-
		(b)	103	-	3	8	11	15	23	21	14	6	2
748	Congenital anomalies of respiratory system	(a)	7	-	1	1	-	2	2	1	-	-	-
		(b)	163	1	7	43	24	28	26	21	4	1	8
749-751	Cleft palate and lip; other congenital anomalies of upper alimentary tract and digestive system	(a)	12	-	-	2	2	3	5	-	-	-	-
		(b)	43	-	2	7	11	4	13	1	4	-	1
753	Congenital anomalies of urinary sustem	(a)	31	-	5	10	9	3	2	1	1	-	-
		(b)	101	-	1	16	23	35	12	8	2	-	4
754-756	Congenital musculoskeletal anomalies	(a)	33	-	5	9	3	7	7	1	1	-	-
		(b)	124	-	4	15	18	29	21	20	7	4	6
758	Chromosomal anomalies	(a)	21	-	5	9	3	2	1	1	-	-	-
		(b)	73	-	4	11	22	15	11	6	3	-	1
740-759 rem	Other and unspecified congenital anomalies	(a)	61	3	14	16	10	7	6	3	-	1	1
		(b)	102	-	10	13	27	24	14	8	4	1	1
764,765	Prematurity	(a)	181	10	57	51	31	22	7	1	-	-	2
		(b)	882	68	566	141	45	10	6	8	3	4	31
764	Slow fetal growth and fetal malnutrition	(a)	147	10	47	38	24	20	7	1	-	-	-
		(b)	12	1	6	3	-	-	-	-	-	1	1
765	Disorders relating to short gestation and unspecified low birthweight	(a)	34	-	10	13	7	2	-	-	-	-	2
		(b)	870	67	560	138	45	10	6	8	3	3	30
7650	Extreme immaturity	(a)	3	-	1	1	-	-	-	-	-	-	1
		(b)	634	59	487	47	6	1	2	6	2	2	22
7651	Other preterm infants	(a)	31	-	9	12	7	2	-	-	-	-	1
		(b)	236	8	73	91	39	9	4	2	1	1	8

Table 27a - *continued*

ICD number	Cause of death		Birthweight (grams)										
			All weights	Under 500	500 - 999	1000 - 1499	1500 - 1999	2000 - 2499	2500 - 2999	3000 - 3499	3500 - 3999	4000 and over	Not stated
767	Birth trauma	(a)	12	-	-	1	1	-	3	3	4	-	-
		(b)	87	-	17	17	9	4	14	13	8	3	2
7670	Subdural and cerebral haemorrhage	(a)	12	-	-	1	1	-	3	3	4	-	-
		(b)	77	-	16	17	8	4	12	10	6	3	1
768	Intrauterine hypoxia and birth asphyxia	(a)	1,135	9	78	151	156	218	195	188	87	49	4
		(b)	325	1	17	14	32	48	46	86	45	20	16
7680	Death from asphyxia or anoxia before onset of labour or at unspecified time	(a)	930	7	78	138	139	185	158	133	56	32	4
		(b)	-	-	-	-	-	-	-	-	-	-	-
7681	Death from asphyxia or anoxia during labour	(a)	205	2	-	13	17	33	37	55	31	17	-
		(b)	-	-	-	-	-	-	-	-	-	-	-
7689	Unspecified birth asphyxia in liveborn infant	(a)	-	-	-	-	-	-	-	-	-	-	-
		(b)	180	-	10	11	22	28	26	47	19	9	8
512,514, 516,518, 519,769, 770	Non-infectious respiratory disorders	(a)	10	-	-	1	2	-	3	3	1	-	-
		(b)	904	7	326	258	107	44	58	34	30	11	29
769	Respiratory distress syndrome	(a)	-	-	-	-	-	-	-	-	-	-	-
		(b)	475	3	187	162	67	15	11	3	3	3	21
770	Other respiratory conditions of fetus and newborn	(a)	10	-	-	1	2	-	3	3	1	-	-
		(b)	426	4	139	96	40	29	47	30	25	8	8
001-139, 320-326, 460-511, 513,771	Infections and infectious diseases	(a)	10	-	2	2	2	1	1	1	-	-	1
		(b)	199	-	25	43	21	31	25	33	13	3	5
320-322	Meningitis	(a)	-	-	-	-	-	-	-	-	-	-	-
		(b)	26	-	1	3	2	6	4	8	2	-	-
480-486	Pneumonia	(a)	-	-	-	-	-	-	-	-	-	-	-
		(b)	47	-	4	5	4	7	6	14	5	1	1
771	Infections specific to the perinatal period	(a)	10	-	2	2	2	1	1	1	-	-	1
		(b)	108	-	19	33	15	14	11	6	4	2	4
766, 772-779	Other perinatal causes	(a)	441	19	43	92	72	59	57	53	24	14	8
		(b)	455	2	139	103	62	34	48	39	17	6	5
766	Disorders relating to long gestation and high birthweight	(a)	9	-	-	-	-	1	1	4	1	2	-
		(b)	3	-	-	-	-	-	-	2	-	1	-
772	Fetal and neonatal haemorrhage	(a)	14	-	-	3	3	1	3	3	-	1	-
		(b)	226	1	101	63	27	4	11	10	4	1	4
773	Haemolytic disease of fetus or newborn, due to isoimmunization	(a)	16	-	-	4	3	3	4	1	1	-	-
		(b)	14	-	3	3	7	-	-	1	-	-	-
7730	Due to Rh isoimmunization	(a)	10	-	-	3	2	1	2	1	1	-	-
		(b)	6	-	1	1	4	-	-	-	-	-	-
774	Other perinatal jaundice	(a)	-	-	-	-	-	-	-	-	-	-	-
		(b)	1	-	-	1	-	-	-	-	-	-	-
775	Endocrine and metabolic disturbances specific to the fetus and newborn	(a)	6	-	-	-	-	-	-	1	5	-	-
		(b)	5	-	-	-	1	1	1	1	-	1	-

Table 27a - *continued*

ICD number	Cause of death		All weights	Under 500	500 - 999	1000 - 1499	1500 - 1999	2000 - 2499	2500 - 2999	3000 - 3499	3500 - 3999	4000 and over	Not stated
7750	Syndrome of 'infant to a diabetic mother'	(a)	6	-	-	-	-	-	-	1	5	-	-
		(b)	-	-	-	-	-	-	-	-	-	-	-
776	Haematological disorders of fetus and newborn	(a)	2	-	-	-	-	-	1	1	-	-	-
		(b)	16	-	7	4	3	-	-	1	1	-	-
777	Perinatal disorders of digestive system	(a)	-	-	-	-	-	-	-	-	-	-	-
		(b)	54	-	16	15	6	6	7	-	4	-	-
778	Conditions involving the integument and temperature regulation of fetus and newborn	(a)	20	-	3	3	6	2	5	-	1	-	-
		(b)	30	-	3	4	6	6	4	5	1	1	-
779	Other and ill-defined conditions originating in the perinatal period	(a)	374	19	40	82	60	52	43	43	16	11	8
		(b)	106	1	9	13	12	17	25	19	7	2	1
7799	Unspecified perinatal conditions	(a)	363	16	40	81	60	49	43	42	16	11	5
		(b)	-	-	-	-	-	-	-	-	-	-	-
4275, 428, 584-586, 780-799, 800-999	Ill-defined conditions, modes of death, injury and poisoning	(a)	2	-	-	-	-	-	1	1	-	-	-
		(b)	153	1	11	10	10	18	23	41	29	7	3
798	Sudden death, cause unknown	(a)	-	-	-	-	-	-	-	-	-	-	-
		(b)	78	-	-	1	2	8	13	29	21	4	-
7980	Sudden infant death syndrome	(a)	-	-	-	-	-	-	-	-	-	-	-
		(b)	78	-	-	1	2	8	13	29	21	4	-
760-763	Maternal conditions certified as fetal	(a)	627	16	86	94	95	107	87	89	29	17	7
		(b)	35	-	11	1	2	5	4	7	3	1	1
001-E999 rem	Other fetal causes	(a)	14	1	3	3	2	1	3	-	1	-	-
		(b)	98	-	7	3	11	17	14	23	15	7	1
7996	No fetal cause	(a)	1,111	18	140	194	138	189	177	148	70	31	6
		(b)	5	-	3	-	-	-	1	-	-	-	1
	Maternal mentions	(a)	1,342	18	158	260	192	249	195	134	87	43	6
		(b)	906	24	351	206	103	58	52	56	19	10	27
642, 7600	Hypertension	(a)	254	5	64	63	31	32	18	22	13	5	1
		(b)	117	3	64	22	8	6	4	5	2	1	2
647,648, 760 rem	Other maternal conditions which may be unrelated to the present pregnancy	(a)	30	1	3	3	3	2	2	5	3	8	-
		(b)	18	1	3	4	3	3	2	1	1	-	-
761	Maternal complications in pregnancy	(a)	-	-	-	-	-	-	-	-	-	-	-
		(b)	1	-	-	-	-	1	-	-	-	-	-
762	Complications of placenta, cord and membranes	(a)	-	-	-	-	-	-	-	-	-	-	-
		(b)	-	-	-	-	-	-	-	-	-	-	-
651, 7615	Multiple pregnancy	(a)	44	3	8	11	13	5	3	-	-	-	1
		(b)	61	2	30	16	6	1	2	-	1	1	2
630-639, 643,646, 650,663, 655-658, 670-676, 761-762 rem	Other maternal complications of pregnancy, placenta, cord or membranes	(a)	333	6	39	59	38	54	61	41	25	8	2
		(b)	232	7	67	66	32	23	13	13	3	-	8

Table 27a - *continued*

ICD number	Cause of death		Birthweight (grams)										
			All weights	Under 500	500 - 999	1000 - 1499	1500 - 1999	2000 - 2499	2500 - 2999	3000 - 3499	3500 - 3999	4000 and over	Not stated
7622	Other and unspecified morphological and functional abnormalities of placenta	(a) (b)	- -	- -	- -	- -	- -	- -	- -	- -	- -	- -	- -
7624	Prolapsed cord	(a) (b)	- -	- -	- -	- -	- -	- -	- -	- -	- -	- -	- -
7625	Other compression of umbilical cord	(a) (b)	- -	- -	- -	- -	- -	- -	- -	- -	- -	- -	- -
640,641, 7620, 7621	Maternal antepartum haemorrhage	(a) (b)	506 180	2 5	26 72	106 36	83 20	128 11	88 10	47 11	19 5	5 3	2 7
7620	Placenta praevia	(a) (b)	- -	- -	- -	- -	- -	- -	- -	- -	- -	- -	- -
7621	Other forms of placental separation and haemorrhage	(a) (b)	- -	- -	- -	- -	- -	- -	- -	- -	- -	- -	- -
644,645, 652-654, 659-662, 664-669, 7610, 7617,763	Complications of presentation, labour and delivery	(a) (b)	45 212	- 4	- 92	5 47	4 18	9 8	5 9	10 20	9 6	3 1	- 7
763	Other complications of labour and delivery	(a) (b)	- 1	- -	- -	- -	- -	- 1	- -	- -	- -	- -	- -
001-E999 rem	Other maternal conditions	(a) (b)	130 86	1 2	18 23	13 15	20 16	19 6	18 12	9 6	18 1	14 4	- 1
7996	No maternal cause	(a) (b)	2,308 2,637	55 57	281 667	376 351	327 263	359 279	345 319	344 354	132 204	67 68	22 75
Total live births		M F P	338,852 322,166 661,018	83 65 148	1,015 902 1,917	2,084 1,932 4,016	4,406 4,488 8,894	14,008 16,745 30,753	52,944 66,866 119,810	122,696 129,339 252,035	102,735 80,379 183,114	38,554 21,153 59,707	327 297 624

Table 27b Stillbirths (a), and neonatal deaths (b) - rates per 1,000 total/live births: birthweight by selected cause of death, 1986　　　　　England and Wales

N - list number	Cause of death		Birthweight (grams)										
			All weights	Under 500	500 - 999	1000 - 1499	1500 - 1999	2000 - 2499	2500 - 2999	3000 - 3499	3500 - 3999	4000 and over	Not stated
	All causes												
	Stillbirth rates	(a)	5.3	327.3	181.8	133.7	53.3	18.8	4.4	1.8	1.2	1.7	42.9
	Neonatal death rates	(b)	5.2	533.8	512.8	132.7	40.1	10.7	3.0	1.6	1.2	1.3	163.5
	Fetal mentions	(a)	4.1	268.2	136.2	101.2	43.2	14.3	3.3	1.4	0.8	1.4	36.8
		(b)	6.6	567.6	603.5	181.8	54.5	14.7	4.0	2.0	1.4	1.7	195.5
N01	Anencephalus	(a)	0.1	4.5	3.8	3.0	1.0	0.1	0.0	-	0.0	0.0	1.5
		(b)	0.0	-	1.6	1.5	0.6	0.2	0.0	0.0	-	-	1.6
N02	Spina bifida	(a)	0.0	-	0.9	0.9	0.1	0.2	0.0	0.0	0.0	-	-
		(b)	0.1	13.5	-	0.7	0.8	0.4	0.2	0.0	0.0	0.0	-
N03	Encephalocele	(a)	0.0	-	-	-	0.1	-	-	-	-	-	-
		(b)	0.0	6.8	-	1.0	0.3	0.2	0.1	0.0	0.0	-	1.6
N04	Other congenital anomalies of central nervous system	(a)	0.1	-	2.6	1.7	0.4	0.1	0.1	0.0	0.0	-	-
		(b)	0.1	-	1.6	0.2	1.7	0.4	0.1	0.0	0.0	0.1	1.6
N05	Congenital anomalies of circulatory system	(a)	0.0	-	1.3	0.2	0.3	0.1	0.0	-	-	0.0	-
		(b)	0.7	6.8	2.1	5.2	3.5	2.3	0.8	0.5	0.4	0.4	8.0
N06	Other congenital anomalies	(a)	0.2	13.6	12.8	10.1	2.9	0.8	0.2	0.0	0.0	0.0	1.5
		(b)	0.9	6.8	14.6	26.1	14.1	4.4	0.8	0.3	0.1	0.1	33.7
N07	Prematurity	(a)	0.3	45.5	24.3	11.0	3.3	0.7	0.1	0.0	-	-	3.1
		(b)	1.3	459.5	295.3	35.1	5.1	0.3	0.1	0.0	0.0	0.1	49.7
N08	Birth trauma	(a)	0.0	-	-	0.2	0.1	-	0.0	0.0	0.0	-	-
		(b)	0.1	-	8.9	4.2	1.0	0.1	0.1	0.1	0.0	0.1	3.2
N09	Birth asphyxia	(a)	1.7	40.9	33.3	32.6	16.6	7.0	1.6	0.7	0.5	0.8	6.1
		(b)	0.5	6.8	8.9	3.5	3.6	1.6	0.4	0.3	0.2	0.3	25.6
N10	Non-infectious respiratory disorders	(a)	0.0	-	-	0.2	0.2	-	0.0	0.0	0.0	-	-
		(b)	1.4	47.3	170.1	64.2	12.0	1.4	0.5	0.1	0.2	0.2	46.5
N11	Infections and infectious diseases	(a)	0.0	-	0.9	0.4	0.2	0.0	0.0	0.0	-	-	1.5
		(b)	0.3	-	13.0	10.7	2.4	1.0	0.2	0.1	0.1	0.1	8.0
N12	Other perinatal causes	(a)	0.7	86.4	18.4	19.8	7.7	1.9	0.5	0.2	0.1	0.2	12.3
		(b)	0.7	13.5	72.5	25.6	7.0	1.1	0.4	0.2	0.1	0.1	8.0
N13	Ill-defined conditions, modes of death, injury and poisoning	(a)	0.0	-	-	-	-	-	0.0	0.0	-	-	-
		(b)	0.2	6.8	5.7	2.5	1.1	0.6	0.2	0.2	0.2	0.1	4.8
N14	Maternal conditions classified as fetal	(a)	0.9	72.7	36.7	20.3	10.1	3.4	0.7	0.4	0.2	0.3	10.7
		(b)	0.1	-	5.7	0.2	0.2	0.2	0.0	0.0	0.0	0.0	1.6
N15	Other fetal causes	(a)	0.0	4.5	1.3	0.6	0.2	0.0	0.0	-	0.0	-	-
		(b)	0.1	-	3.7	0.7	1.2	0.6	0.1	0.1	0.1	0.1	1.6
N16	No fetal cause	(a)	1.7	81.8	59.8	41.8	14.7	6.0	1.5	0.6	0.4	0.5	9.2
		(b)	0.0	-	1.6	-	-	-	0.0	-	-	-	1.6
	Maternal mentions	(a)	2.0	81.8	67.4	56.1	20.4	7.9	1.6	0.5	0.5	0.7	9.2
		(b)	1.4	162.2	183.1	51.3	11.6	1.9	0.4	0.2	0.1	0.2	43.3
N17	Hypertension	(a)	0.4	22.7	27.3	13.6	3.3	1.0	0.1	0.1	0.1	0.1	1.5
		(b)	0.2	20.3	33.4	5.5	0.9	0.2	0.0	0.0	0.0	0.0	3.2
N18	Other maternal conditions which may be unrelated to the present pregnancy	(a)	0.0	4.5	1.3	0.6	0.3	0.1	0.0	0.0	0.0	0.1	-
		(b)	0.0	6.8	1.6	1.0	0.3	0.1	0.0	0.0	0.0	-	-
N19	Multiple pregnancy	(a)	0.1	13.6	3.4	2.4	1.4	0.2	0.0	-	-	-	1.5
		(b)	0.1	13.5	15.6	4.0	0.7	0.0	0.0	-	0.0	0.0	3.2

Table 27b - *continued*

N - list number	Cause of death		Birthweight (grams)										
			All weights	Under 500	500 - 999	1000 - 1499	1500 - 1999	2000 - 2499	2500 - 2999	3000 - 3499	3500 - 3999	4000 and over	Not stated
N20	Other maternal complications related to pregnancy, placenta, cord or membranes	(a)	0.5	27.3	16.6	12.7	4.0	1.7	0.5	0.2	0.1	0.1	3.1
		(b)	0.4	47.3	35.0	16.4	3.6	0.7	0.1	0.1	0.0	-	12.8
N21	Maternal antepartum haemorrhage	(a)	0.8	9.1	11.1	22.9	8.8	4.1	0.7	0.2	0.1	0.1	3.1
		(b)	0.3	33.8	37.6	9.0	2.2	0.4	0.1	0.0	0.0	0.1	11.2
N22	Complications of presentation, labour and delivery	(a)	0.1	-	-	1.1	0.4	0.3	0.0	0.0	0.0	0.1	-
		(b)	0.3	27.0	48.0	11.7	2.0	0.3	0.1	0.1	0.0	0.0	11.2
N23	Other maternal conditions	(a)	0.2	4.5	7.7	2.8	2.0	0.6	0.1	0.0	0.1	0.2	-
		(b)	0.1	13.5	12.0	3.7	1.8	0.2	0.1	0.0	0.0	0.1	1.6
N24	No maternal cause	(a)	3.5	250.0	119.9	81.1	34.8	11.5	2.9	1.4	0.7	1.1	33.7
		(b)	4.0	385.1	347.9	87.4	29.6	9.1	2.7	1.4	1.1	1.1	120.2

Table 28 Postneonatal deaths - numbers and rates per 1,000 live births : England and Wales
birthweight by selected underlying cause of death, 1986

ICD	Cause of death	Birthweight (grams)										
		All weights	Under 500	500-999	1000-1499	1500-1999	2000-2499	2500-2999	3000-3499	3500-3999	4000 and over	Not stated
	Numbers											
	All causes	2,760	3	119	122	186	276	591	816	490	146	11
001-139	**I Infectious and parasitic diseases**	98	-	6	5	5	11	23	28	15	5	-
460-519	**VIII Diseases of the respiratory system**	306	-	5	6	20	34	61	98	63	18	1
460-465	Diseases of upper respiratory tract	27	-	-	-	1	3	6	10	5	2	-
466	Acute bronchitis and bronchiolitis	87	-	-	1	7	9	8	34	22	5	1
480-486	Pneumonia	129	-	1	2	8	16	29	41	24	8	-
740-759	**XIV Congenital anomalies**	465	-	6	14	47	82	118	119	58	18	3
740	Anencephalus and similar anomalies	1	-	-	-	-	1	-	-	-	-	-
741	Spina bifida	42	-	-	-	2	7	12	11	9	1	-
742	Other congenital anomalies of nervous system	45	-	1	1	4	8	14	10	3	4	-
745-747	Congenital anomalies of heart and circulatory system	263	-	3	4	16	42	67	77	42	11	1
760-779	**XV Certain conditions originating in the perinatal period**	202	3	84	54	14	5	12	14	7	2	7
798	Sudden death, cause unknown	1,284	-	11	31	72	96	292	438	272	72	-
E800-E999	**EXVII External causes of injury and poisoning**	94	-	2	4	3	10	19	33	16	7	-
E911	Inhalation and ingestion of food causing obstruction of respiratory tract or suffocation	30	-	1	2	-	2	9	10	5	1	-
E913	Accidental mechanical suffocation	11	-	-	1	1	1	2	3	1	2	-
	Rates											
	All causes	4.2	17.2	62.1	30.4	20.9	9.0	4.9	3.2	2.7	2.4	17.6
001-139	**I Infectious and parasitic diseases**	0.1	-	3.1	1.2	0.6	0.4	0.2	0.1	0.1	0.1	-
460-519	**VIII Diseases of the respiratory system**	0.5	-	2.6	1.5	2.2	1.1	0.5	0.4	0.3	0.3	1.6
460-465	Diseases of upper respiratory tract	0.0	-	-	-	0.1	0.1	0.1	0.0	0.0	0.0	-
466	Acute bronchitis and bronchiolitis	0.1	-	-	0.2	0.8	0.3	0.1	0.1	0.1	0.1	1.6
480-486	Pneumonia	0.2	-	0.5	0.5	0.9	0.5	0.2	0.2	0.1	0.1	-
740-759	**XIV Congenital anomalies**	0.7	-	3.1	3.5	5.3	2.7	1.0	0.5	0.3	0.3	4.8
740	Anencephalus and similar anomalies	0.0	-	-	-	-	0.0	-	-	-	-	-
741	Spina bifida	0.1	-	-	-	0.2	0.2	0.1	0.0	0.0	0.0	-
742	Other congenital anomalies of nervous system	0.1	-	0.5	0.2	0.4	0.3	0.1	0.0	0.0	0.1	-
745-747	Congenital anomalies of heart and circulatory system	0.4	-	1.6	1.0	1.8	1.4	0.6	0.3	0.2	0.2	1.6
760-779	**XV Certain conditions originating in the perinatal period**	0.3	17.2	43.8	13.4	1.6	0.2	0.1	0.1	0.0	0.0	11.2
798	Sudden death, cause unknown	1.9	-	5.7	7.7	8.1	3.1	2.4	1.7	1.5	1.2	-
E800-E999	**EXVII External causes of injury and poisoning**	0.1	-	1.0	1.0	0.3	0.3	0.2	0.1	0.1	0.1	-
E911	Inhalation and ingestion of food causing obstruction of respiratory tract or suffocation	0.0	-	0.5	0.5	-	0.1	0.1	0.0	0.0	0.0	-
E913	Accidental mechanical suffocation	0.0	-	-	0.2	0.1	0.0	0.0	0.0	0.0	0.0	-

Table 29a Neonatal deaths - numbers and rates per 1,000 live births: age of mother by place of confinement and legitimacy, 1986

England and Wales

Place of confinement	Legitimacy	Age of mother											
		All ages		Under 20		20-24		25-29		30-34		35 and over	
		Number	Rate	Number	Rate	Number	Rate	Number	Rate	Number	Rate	Number	Rate
All	All	3,449	5.2	435	7.6	1,009	5.3	1,074	4.7	597	4.6	334	6.3
	Legitimate	2,461	4.7	103	5.8	645	4.7	917	4.6	519	4.5	277	6.0
	Illegitimate	988	7.0	332	8.4	364	6.7	157	5.7	78	5.9	57	8.4
NHS hospital A	All	24	1.6	3	3.8	6	1.4	5	0.8	7	2.3	3	4.5
	Legitimate	19	1.5	2	6.9	3	0.9	5	0.9	6	2.1	3	4.9
	Illegitimate	5	2.4	1	2.0	3	3.4	-	-	1	4.7	-	-
NHS hospital B	All	3,337	5.3	414	7.4	981	5.3	1,053	4.8	572	4.7	317	6.2
	Legitimate	2,383	4.8	97	5.6	627	4.8	900	4.7	498	4.5	261	5.9
	Illegitimate	954	6.9	317	8.2	354	6.7	153	5.7	74	5.9	56	8.5
Other hospital	All	20	2.7	1	3.7	5	2.5	4	1.7	6	3.5	4	4.6
	Legitimate	19	2.8	1	5.6	5	2.6	3	1.3	6	3.7	4	4.9
	Illegitimate	1	2.2	-	-	-	-	1	10.8	-	-	-	-
At home	All	55	9.2	16	58.2	13	11.5	9	4.1	9	5.2	8	11.7
	Legitimate	32	6.9	2	35.7	9	11.6	7	3.9	7	4.7	7	12.7
	Illegitimate	23	17.2	14	63.9	4	11.2	2	5.3	2	7.7	1	7.8
Elsewhere	All	13	24.6	1	16.7	4	25.2	3	17.3	3	32.6	2	45.5
	Legitimate	8	24.4	1	62.5	1	11.9	2	16.7	2	28.6	2	52.6
	Illegitimate	5	25.0	-	-	3	40.0	1	18.9	1	45.5	-	-

Table 29b Live births - numbers: age of mother by place of confinement and legitimacy, 1986

England and Wales

Place of confinement	Legitimacy	Age of mother					
		All ages	Under 20	20-24	25-29	30-34	35 and over
All	All	661,018	57,406	192,064	229,035	129,487	53,026
	Legitimate	519,673	17,793	137,985	201,323	116,369	46,203
	Illegitimate	141,345	39,613	54,079	27,712	13,118	6,823
NHS hospital A	All	14,892	783	4,374	6,049	3,019	667
	Legitimate	12,828	290	3,494	5,625	2,806	613
	Illegitimate	2,064	493	880	424	213	54
NHS hospital B	All	632,309	56,018	184,368	218,221	122,939	50,763
	Legitimate	495,012	17,253	131,742	191,454	110,379	44,184
	Illegitimate	137,297	38,765	52,626	26,767	12,560	6,579
Other hospital	All	7,283	270	2,032	2,413	1,697	871
	Legitimate	6,838	178	1,890	2,320	1,634	816
	Illegitimate	445	92	142	93	63	55
At home	All	6,006	275	1,131	2,179	1,740	681
	Legitimate	4,667	56	775	1,804	1,480	552
	Illegitimate	1,339	219	356	375	260	129
Elsewhere	All	528	60	159	173	92	44
	Legitimate	328	16	84	120	70	38
	Illegitimate	200	44	75	53	22	6

Table 30 Live births, stillbirths and infant deaths occurring among children born in England and Wales
1985 - numbers and rates per 1,000 total/live births: month of birth, 1985

Note: Children in this table all born in same year, but death may have occurred in that year or following year.

Year of birth	Month of birth	Live births	Stillbirths	Early neonatal deaths	Late neonatal deaths	Postneonatal deaths	Infant deaths
	Numbers						
1985	January	54,707	310	222	62	211	495
	February	49,640	261	191	50	175	416
	March	56,047	320	234	62	179	475
	April	53,262	302	265	50	166	481
	May	57,544	331	237	51	195	483
	June	54,455	289	241	52	211	504
	July	58,188	333	267	61	252	580
	August	57,106	332	241	41	289	571
	September	56,974	318	236	62	274	572
	October	55,843	283	248	57	265	570
	November	51,906	277	222	66	247	535
	December	50,745	289	213	52	224	489
	Total	**656,417**	**3,645**	**2,817**	**666**	**2,688**	**6,171**
	Rates						
	January		5.6	4.1	1.1	3.9	9.0
	February		5.2	3.8	1.0	3.5	8.4
	March		5.7	4.2	1.1	3.2	8.5
	April		5.6	5.0	0.9	3.1	9.0
	May		5.7	4.1	0.9	3.4	8.4
	June		5.3	4.4	1.0	3.9	9.3
	July		5.7	4.6	1.0	4.3	10.0
	August		5.8	4.2	0.7	5.1	10.0
	September		5.6	4.1	1.1	4.8	10.0
	October		5.0	4.4	1.0	4.7	10.2
	November		5.3	4.3	1.3	4.8	10.3
	December		5.7	4.2	1.0	4.4	9.6
	Total		**5.5**	**4.3**	**1.0**	**4.1**	**9.4**

Table 31 Stillbirths, infant deaths and live births - numbers and rates per 1,000 total/live births: birthweight by multiplicity, 1985

Multiplicity	Birthweight (grams)	Stillbirths		Early neonatal deaths		Late neonatal deaths		Postneonatal deaths		Infant deaths		Live births
		Number	Rate	Number	Rate	Number	Rate	Number	Rate	Number	Rate	Number
Singleton	**All weights**	**3,405**	**5.3**	**2,486**	**3.9**	**616**	**1.0**	**2,540**	**4.0**	**5,642**	**8.8**	642,934
	Under 2,500	2,043	51.5	1,634	43.4	267	7.1	584	15.5	2,485	66.0	37,629
	Under 1,500	972	168.0	1,110	230.7	153	31.8	192	39.9	1,455	302.4	4,812
	1,500-1,999	531	73.8	241	36.2	39	5.9	140	21.0	420	63.0	6,664
	2,000-2,499	540	20.2	283	10.8	75	2.9	252	9.6	610	23.3	26,153
	2,500-2,999	546	4.7	278	2.4	111	1.0	543	4.7	932	8.0	115,999
	3,000-3,499	463	1.8	262	1.0	128	0.5	804	3.2	1,194	4.8	249,954
	3,500 and over	301	1.3	200	0.8	98	0.4	601	2.5	899	3.8	238,507
	Not stated	52	58.0	112	132.5	12	14.2	8	9.5	132	156.2	845
Multiple	**All weights**	**240**	**17.5**	**331**	**24.5**	**50**	**3.7**	**148**	**11.0**	**529**	**39.2**	13,483
	Under 2,500	193	26.7	302	42.9	44	6.3	118	16.8	464	66.0	7,035
	Under 1,500	106	88.8	253	232.5	30	27.6	42	38.6	325	298.7	1,088
	1,500-1,999	52	26.7	34	18.0	10	5.3	29	15.3	73	38.6	1,892
	2,000-2,499	35	8.6	15	3.7	4	1.0	47	11.6	66	16.3	4,055
	2,500-2,999	30	6.7	15	3.4	3	0.7	20	4.5	38	8.5	4,464
	3,000-3,499	8	4.7	5	2.9	-	-	8	4.7	13	7.7	1,699
	3,500 and over	1	3.8	-	-	-	-	1	3.8	1	3.8	262
	Not stated	8	258.1	9	391.3	3	130.4	1	43.5	13	565.2	23

Table 32 Multiple Births in 1985 - numbers and rates per 1,000 total/live births by live births, stillbirths and infant deaths

	All multiple births		All twin births								Other multiple births	
			All twins		Two males		One male one female		Two females			
	Number	Rate	Number	Rate	Number	Rate	Number	Rate	Number	Rate	Number	Rate
Live births	**13,483**		13,168		4,637		3,816		4,715		315	
Stillbirths	**240**	**17.5**	232	17.3	113	23.8	34	8.8	85	17.7	8	24.8
Early neonatal deaths	**331**	**24.5**	318	24.1	118	25.4	74	19.4	126	26.7	13	41.3
Late neonatal deaths	**50**	**3.7**	45	3.4	16	3.5	16	4.2	13	2.8	5	15.9
Postneonatal deaths	**148**	**11.0**	141	10.7	59	12.7	45	11.8	37	7.8	7	22.2
Infant deaths	**529**	**39.2**	504	38.3	193	41.6	135	35.4	176	37.3	25	79.4

Appendix A N-list numbers and associated ICD codes

N-list number	Description	ICD number
	Fetal Mentions	
N01	Anencephalus	740
N02	Spina bifida	741
N03	Encephalocele	742.0
N04	Other congenital anomalies of central nervous system	742 rem
N05	Congenital anomalies of circulatory system	745-747
N06	Other congenital anomalies	740-759 rem
N07	Prematurity	764, 765
N08	Birth trauma	767
N09	Birth asphyxia	768
N10	Non-infectious respiratory disorders	512, 514, 516, 518, 519, 769, 770
N11	Infections and infectious diseases	001-139, 320-326, 460-511, 513, 771
N12	Other perinatal causes	766, 772-779
N13	Ill-defined conditions, modes of death, injury and poisoning	427.5, 428, 584-586, 780-799, 800-999
N14	Maternal conditions classified as fetal	760-763
N15	Other fetal causes	001-E999 rem
N16	No fetal cause	799.6
	Maternal mentions	
N17	Hypertension	642, 760.0
N18	Other maternal conditions which may be unrelated to the present pregnancy	647, 648, 760 rem
N19	Multiple pregnancy	651, 761.5
N20	Other maternal complications related to pregnancy, placenta, cord or membranes	630-639, 643, 646, 650, 655-658, 663, 670-676, 761-762 rem
N21	Maternal antepartum haemorrhage	640, 641, 762.0, 762.1
N22	Complications of presentation, labour and delivery	644, 645, 652-654, 659-662, 664-669, 761.0, 761.7, 763
N23	Other maternal conditions	001-E999 rem
N24	No maternal cause	799.6

Printed in the United Kingdom for Her Majesty's Stationery Office
C8 12/88

OPCS reference series

OPCS produce a wide range of reference volumes; most of these are annual series which greatly expand on the summary statistics to be found in the related OPCS Monitor series, others appear less frequently as the data becomes available.

Series DH   **Deaths**

DH1	Mortality statistics
DH2	Mortality statistics: cause
DH3	Mortality statistics: perinatal and infant (social and biological factors)
DH4	Mortality statistics: accidents and violence
DH5	Mortality statistics: area
DH6	Mortality statistics: childhood

Series FM   **Family statistics**

FM1	Birth statistics
FM2	Marriage and divorce statistics

Series MB   **Morbidity**

MB1	Cancer statistics
MB2	Communicable disease statistics
MB3	Congenital malformation statistics
MB4	Hospital in-patient statistics (no publications after spring 1989)
MB5	Morbidity statistics from general practice

Series PP   **Population estimates and projections**

PP1	Key population and vital statistics: local and health authority areas
PP2	Population projections - national figures
PP3	Population projections - sub-national figures

Series AB   **Abortion statistics**

Series DR   **Demographic Review**

Series DS   **Decennial supplement** (topics covered include occupational mortality, childhood mortality, area mortality, immigrant mortality, and English life tables)

Series EL   **Electoral statistics**

Series GHS   **General Household Survey**

Series LFS   **Labour Force Survey**

Series LS   **Longitudinal Study** (occasional reports on a range of social and medical subjects)

Series MN   **International migration**

All OPCS reference series are published by HMSO and are available from:

HMSO Publications Centre
(Mail and telephone orders only)
PO Box 276, London, SW8 5DT
Telephone orders (01) 873 9090
General enquiries (01) 873 0011
Standing orders (01) 211 0363

HMSO Bookshops

HMSO's accredited agents
and through good booksellers